INTRODUCTION TO EEG- AND SPEECH-BASED EMOTION RECOGNITION

INTRODUCTION TO EEG- AND SPEECH-BASED EMOTION RECOGNITION

PRIYANKA A. ABHANG
BHARTI W. GAWALI
SURESH C. MEHROTRA

Department of Computer Science and Information Technology,
Dr. Babasaheb Ambedkar Marathwada University, Aurangabad, India

ELSEVIER

AMSTERDAM • BOSTON • HEIDELBERG • LONDON
NEW YORK • OXFORD • PARIS • SAN DIEGO
SAN FRANCISCO • SINGAPORE • SYDNEY • TOKYO

Academic Press is an imprint of Elsevier

Academic Press is an imprint of Elsevier
125 London Wall, London EC2Y 5AS, UK
525 B Street, Suite 1800, San Diego, CA 92101-4495, USA
50 Hampshire Street, 5th Floor, Cambridge, MA 02139, USA
The Boulevard, Langford Lane, Kidlington, Oxford OX5 1GB, UK

British Library Cataloguing-in-Publication Data
A catalogue record for this book is available from the British Library

Library of Congress Cataloging-in-Publication Data
A catalog record for this book is available from the Library of Congress

ISBN: 978-0-12-804490-2

For information on all Academic Press publications
visit our website at https://www.elsevier.com/

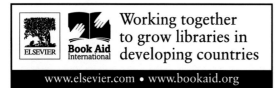

Working together
to grow libraries in
developing countries

www.elsevier.com • www.bookaid.org

Publisher: Mara Conner
Acquisition Editor: Natalie Farra
Editorial Project Manager: Kristi Anderson
Production Project Manager: Edward Taylor
Designer: Mark Rogers

Typeset by TNQ Books and Journals
www.tnq.co.in

Contents

Preface

The human brain is the most complex organ. It controls intelligence, senses, body movements, and behavior. The brain is an association of many parts which work in coordination with each other but are functionally unique and special. It is the place where emotions are generated and controlled. Emotions play an important role, as they unite us irrespective of our country, caste or creed. Humans use different ways — speech, face, gesture, and text — to understand and recognize emotions.

This book provides a far-reaching examination of research with different modalities of emotion recognition. The discussion of key topics starts with the physiology of the brain, followed by brain rhythms, speech parameters, acquisition and analysis tools, features of the modalities, and a case study. It concludes with applications for brain—computer interfacing.

A special feature of this book lies in its inclusion of two very important modalities of emotion: electroencephalography (EEG) signals/images and speech signals, used together. It also presents features to be considered when researchers experiment with recognition with different modalities.

It is hoped that this introduction to EEG- and speech-based emotion recognition will be of great interest to young researchers and postgraduate students. It provides basic knowledge regarding the domain, and focuses on various computational techniques to be implemented. It proposes many research problems to young researchers to prepare them for their own research.

Emotion recognition has been proven to be a significant research area which will be important in designing and developing human—computer interface systems. The material provided in this book is referenced for further reading, and is presented in eight chapters.

Chapter 1, "Introduction to Emotion, Electroencephalography, and Speech Processing" outlines the fundamental aspects of the book's theme. It introduces the basic aspects of the physiology of the brain, EEG, the human auditory system, and speech emotion recognition.

Chapter 2, "Technological Basics of EEG Recording and Operation of Apparatus" presents technological basics of EEG and speech. It gives details of EEG and speech acquisition tools, and describes the Acquire and Analysis software available with the equipment.

Chapter 3, "Technical Aspects of Brain Rhythms and Speech Parameters" introduces brain frequencies along with the speech features considered during analysis. It also explains the preprocessing, feature extraction, and classification techniques which can be implemented in emotion recognition research.

The data acquired through EEG and computerized speech laboratories is in the frequency and time domains. Chapter 4, "Time and Frequency Analysis" illuminates mathematical techniques related to time and frequency analysis transformation. It also provides examples related to the transformation described in the chapter.

Chapter 5, "Emotion Recognition" sheds light on modalities researched in emotion recognition systems. Modalities like face, gesture, speech, text, and brain imaging are individually explained, along with their features.

To recognize emotion properly, much information is needed, along with the tone of speech, how the face looks and how gestures are used add to the recognition of emotion. This information raises the concept of multimodality. Chapter 6, "Multimodal Emotion Recognition" explains the concept of multimodal emotion recognition, and different models and theories of emotion. It also reviews the earlier efforts in multimodal emotion recognition systems, and provides information about online databases available for multimodal emotions. The chapter concludes by discussing challenges for these systems.

Chapter 7, "Proposed EEG/Speech-Based Emotion Recognition System: A Case Study" outlines a case study of an EEG/ speech-based emotion recognition experiment with volunteers from the Department of Computer Science and IT, Dr. Babasaheb Ambedkar Marathwada University. The experimental analysis for happy and sad emotional states is discussed. EEG brain images and speech signals are explored in the chapter. Features considered for the analysis and its numeric data are also described. The correlation between the modalities is justified with linear discriminate analysis classification.

The ultimate goal of emotion recognition is to utilize it for the human (brain) and computer interfacing. Chapter 8, "Brain– Computer Interface Systems and Their Applications" discusses the types and applications of brain–computer interfacing, and also highlights the challenges.

We hope that this book will not only be a useful reference source of information for the scientific community, but will also be of help to the general community interested in the subject.

Priyanka A. Abhang
Bharti W. Gawali
Suresh C. Mehrotra

Acknowledgments

We would like to thank all the people who were directly and indirectly involved in supporting us in the accomplishment of this book, and to express our sincere gratitude to all of them.

Firstly, we would like to acknowledge the System Communication and Machine Learning Research Laboratory for all their fundamental support.

A colossal thanks to our youthful and energetic research colleagues Ganesh Manza, Ganesh Janvale, Rakesh Deore, Santosh Gaikwad, Shashibala Rao, Kavita Waghmare, Sangramsing Kayte, Reena Chaudhary, and Arshiya Khan, who have always been full of life and willing to help in the preparation of technical and nontechnical preliminary materials related to the book.

We would like to thank all the authors of the references cited in the book.

We would like to express our thanks to the management of Elsevier, our publishers, for their guidance in various administrative matters related to the book.

Lastly, we would like to thank all our family members for their support throughout the writing of the book.

Priyanka A. Abhang
Bharti W. Gawali
Suresh C. Mehrotra

CHAPTER

1

Introduction to Emotion, Electroencephalography, and Speech Processing

1.1 INTRODUCTION

In a very real sense, we have two minds, one that thinks and one that feels. *Daniel Goleman, Emotional Intelligence.*

Emotions are intrinsically connected to the way that people interact with each other. Emotion constitutes a major influence for determining human behaviors. A human being can read the emotional state of another human, and behave in the best way to improve their communication at that moment. This is because emotions can be recognized through words, voice intonation, facial expression, and body language.

Emotions have been studied in scientific disciplines such as physiology, psychology, speech science, neuroscience, psychiatry, communication, and so on. As a result, distinctive perspectives on the concept of emotions have emerged, appropriate to the complexity and variety of emotions. It is important to see these different perspectives as complementary to each other.

In humans, emotions fundamentally involve physiological arousal, expressive behaviors, and conscious experience. Thus in that respect there are three views of emotions.

- Psychological (what one is thinking).
- Physiological (what one's body is doing).
- Expressive (how one reacts) in nature.

It is thought that emotions are predictable, and are settled in the different regions in the brain depending on what emotion is invoked. An emotional reaction can be separated into three major categories: behavioral, automatic, and hormonal.[1]

In psychology, expression of emotion is viewed as a reaction to stimuli that involves characteristic physiological changes. According to psychology, an emotion is seen as a disturbance in the homeostatic baseline. Based on these changes, the properties of emotions can be represented as a three-dimensional construct. Essential dimensions of emotional states are measured by the features of activation.

- Arousal: measured as an intensity.
- Affect: valence of pressure, measured as positive or negative feeling after emotion perception.
- Power (control): measured as dominance or submissiveness in emotion expression.

Thus the psychology of emotions can be viewed as a complex experience of consciousness (psychology), bodily sensation (physiology), and behavior (active speech). Orientational dimensions of emotional states are captured by the features of activation, affection, and power.

The emotions generally represent a synthesis of subjective experience, expressive behavior, and neurochemical activity. In the physiology of emotion production mechanisms, it has been found that the nervous system is stimulated by the expression of high-arousal emotions such as anger, happiness, and fear. This phenomenon causes an increased heart rate, higher blood pressure, changes in respiratory pattern, greater subglottal air pressure in the lungs, and dryness in the mouth.[2]

Emotions are generally expressed in positive and negative ways. The positive emotions such as happiness, excitement, joy, etc. are pleasant and are seen as constructive in an individual, whereas negative emotions such as sadness, anger, fear, etc. are considered unpleasant and may be considered to be destructive for an individual.

According to Robert Plutchik,[3] any emotion is based upon one of six primary emotions. Happiness, sadness, anger, disgust, fear, and surprise are considered as the main or basic emotions by most researchers and are known as archetypal emotions.[4]

1. **Happiness** is the emotion that expresses various degrees of positive feelings, ranging from satisfaction to extreme joy.

2. **Sadness** is the emotion that expresses a state of loss or difficulty. Sadness causes individuals to be slow at processing information.
3. **Anger** is the emotion that expresses dislike or opposition toward a person or thing that is causing aversion. Anger is sometimes displayed through sudden and overt aggressive acts.
4. **Disgust** is the emotion that expresses a reaction to things that are considered dirty, revolting, contagious, contaminated, or inedible. Disgust is associated with a distinct facial expression and a drop in heart rate.
5. **Fear** is the emotional reaction to an actual and specific source of danger. Fear is often confused with anxiety, which is an emotion that is often exaggerated and experienced even when the source of danger is not present or tangible.
6. **Surprise** is the emotion that arises when an individual comes across an unanticipated situation. A surprise emotion can be a positive, neutral, or negative experience. A human being can understand the emotional state of another human being and behave in the best manner to improve the communication in a certain situation. This is because emotions can be recognized through various modalities such as words, voice intonation, facial expression, body language and by brain signals.[5]

1.2 BRAIN PHYSIOLOGY

The brain is the central controlling organ of the human being. Various scientific studies have proved that some regions of the brain are involved in thinking of emotions, responding to extreme emotional stimuli, and viewing emotional situations. Nearly all vital activities necessary for survival, as well as all emotions, originate inside the brain. The brain also receives and interprets a multitude of signals sent to it by other parts of the body and the environment.

1.2.1 Major Brain Areas

The brain is composed of a number of different regions, each with specialized functions. Fig. 1.1 shows the major parts of the brain.

The central core of the brain is made up of the brain stem and midbrain. The cerebral cortex is a covering layer for this central core. The central nucleus is moderately elementary and older, and its activity is mainly unconscious. In contrast, the cerebral cortex is extremely developed and capable of deliberation and functions, while the older parts of the brain remain relatively stable.[6]

The Brain Stem

The stem is in between the spinal cord and the rest of the brain. It is made up of the medulla that controls breathing, heart rate, and digestion, and the cerebellum which coordinates sensory input with muscle movement. The functions of the brain stem govern respiration, blood pressure, and some reflexes. The brain stem is further distributed into several distinct sections: the midbrain, pons, and medulla oblongata.

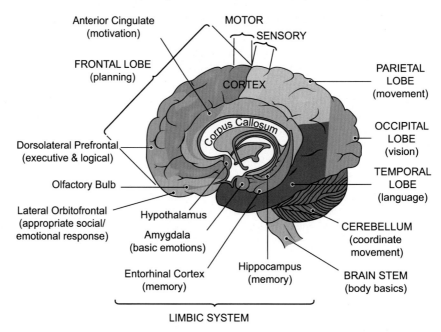

FIGURE 1.1   Major parts of the brain.

The Midbrain

The midbrain consists of features that are intimately connected to human emotion and the shaping of long-term memory via neural connections to the lobes of the cortex. The structures contained also link the lower brain stem to the thalamus to relay information from the senses to the brain, and back out to muscles and the limbic system.

The Limbic System

The limbic system holds the hypothalamus, amygdala, and hippocampus.

- The hypothalamus is responsible for driving actions.
- The amygdala is connected to aggressive behavior.
- The hippocampus plays a crucial role in processing various types of information to form long-term memories.

One key feature of the midbrain and limbic system is the reticular activating system (RAS). It is this area that keeps us awake and aware of the world. The RAS acts as a master switch that alerts the brain to incoming data—and to the urgency of the message.

The Cerebral Cortex

This is the outermost layer of the brain and is the starting point of thinking and voluntary monuments. In humans, the cerebral cortex has evolved into two symmetrical cerebral hemispheres.

The Basal Ganglia

The basal ganglia is a cluster of structures in the center of the brain that coordinates messages between multiple brain regions.

The Cerebellum

The cerebellum is below and behind the cerebrum, at the base and back of the brain, and is tied to the brain stem. It controls motor function and the body's ability to interpret information sent to the brain by the eyes, ears, and other sensory organs. It is responsible for coordination and balance. It is separated into right and left hemispheres; the functions of these are shown in Fig. 1.2.[7]

The brain is divided down the middle into two symmetrical and equal parts, considered as right and left hemispheres. Although equal in size, these two sides are not the same and do not carry out the same functions. Both hemispheres are connected by the corpus callosum and serve the body in different ways.

1. Functions of the left brain.
   a. The left side of the brain is responsible for controlling the right side of the body.
   b. It also performs logical tasks such as those found in science and mathematics.
   c. The left hemisphere is dominant in language.
   d. The left hemisphere is important for preprocessing social emotions.
2. Functions of the right brain.
   a. The right hemisphere is responsible for controlling the left side of the body.
   b. It is responsible for creative awareness.
   c. The right hemisphere is dominant in emotional expression.
   d. It is also dominant in the perception of facial expression, body posture, and prosody.

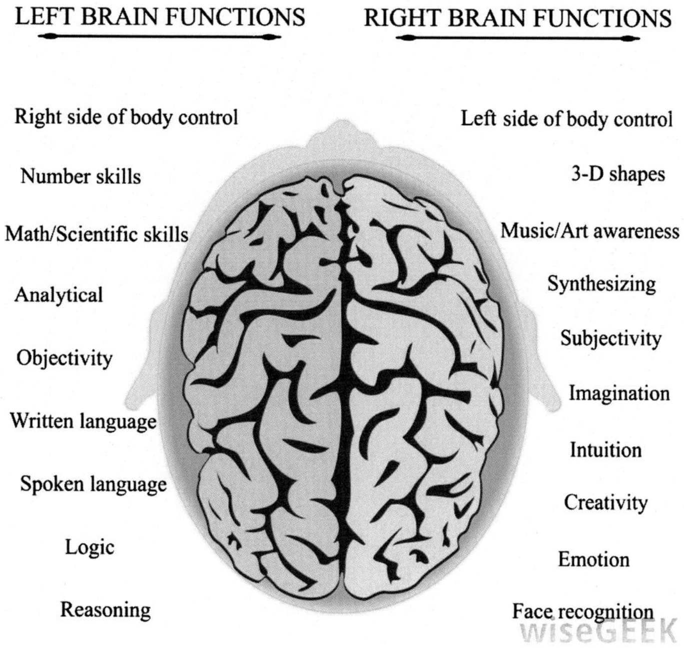

LEFT BRAIN FUNCTIONS   RIGHT BRAIN FUNCTIONS

Right side of body control   Left side of body control

Number skills   3-D shapes

Math/Scientific skills   Music/Art awareness

Analytical   Synthesizing

Objectivity   Subjectivity

Imagination

Written language   Intuition

Spoken language   Creativity

Logic   Emotion

Reasoning   Face recognition

FIGURE 1.2   Functions of left and right hemispheres of the brain.

The Cerebrum

The cerebrum is the largest part of the brain. It is responsible for memory, speech, the senses, and emotional response. It is divided into four sections called lobes: the frontal, temporal, parietal, and occipital. Each handles a specific segment of the cerebrum's jobs.

The diencephalon is inside the cerebrum above the brain stem. Its tasks include sensory function, food intake control, and the body's sleep cycle. As with the other parts of the brain, it is divided into sections. These include the thalamus, hypothalamus, and epitheliums.

The brain is protected from damage by several layers of defenses. Outermost are the bones of the skull. Beneath the skull are the meninges, a series of sturdy membranes that surround the brain and spinal cord. Inside the meninges, the brain is cushioned by fluid.[8]

1.3 LOBES OF THE BRAIN AND THEIR FUNCTIONS

The brain is the most complex organ in the human body. It comprises the frontal, occipital, temporal, and parietal lobes, as shown in Fig. 1.3.

The four lobes have different locations and functions that support the responses and actions of the human body.

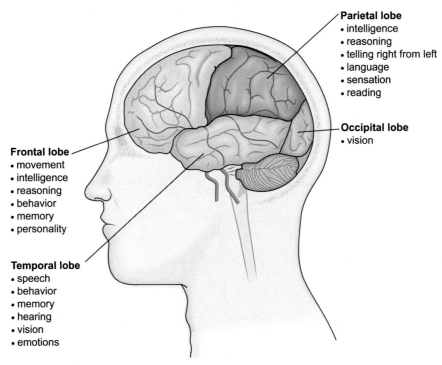

Parietal lobe
- intelligence
- reasoning
- telling right from left
- language
- sensation
- reading

Occipital lobe
- vision

Frontal lobe
- movement
- intelligence
- reasoning
- behavior
- memory
- personality

Temporal lobe
- speech
- behavior
- memory
- hearing
- vision
- emotions

FIGURE 1.3   Different lobes of the brain with their characteristics.

1.3.1 The Frontal Lobe

The *frontal lobe* is the emotional control center of the brain, responsible for forming our personality and influencing out decisions. It is located at the front of the central sulcus, where it receives information signals from other lobes of the brain. The frontal lobe is responsible for problem solving, judgment, and motor function; it controls thinking, planning, organizing, short-term memory, and movement. Most of its functions center on regulating social behavior. Some of the important functions of the frontal lobe include

- cognition, problem solving, and reasoning
- motor skill development
- parts of speech
- impulse control
- spontaneity
- regulating emotions
- regulating sexual urges
- planning.

1.3.2 The Parietal Lobe

The *parietal lobe* processes sensory information for cognitive purposes and helps coordinate spatial relations. It resides in the middle section of the brain behind the central sulcus, above the occipital lobe. The parietal lobe is responsible to manage sensation, handwriting, and body position. It interprets sensory information, such as temperature and touch, and is responsible for processing sensory information from various parts of the body. Some of the functions of the parietal lobe include

- sensing pain, pressure, and touch
- regulating and processing the body's five senses
- movement and visual orientation
- speech
- visual perception and recognition
- cognition and information processing.

1.3.3 The Temporal Lobe

The *temporal lobe* is located at the bottom of the brain below the lateral fissure; there is one temporal lobe on each side of the brain, in close proximity to the ears. This lobe is the location of the primary auditory cortex, which is important for interpreting the sounds and language we hear. The temporal lobes are involved with memory and hearing, and process information from our senses of smell, taste, and sound. They also play a role in memory storage. The primary function of the temporal lobes is to process auditory sounds. Other functions include

- help in formation of long-term memories and processing new information
- formation of visual and verbal memories
- interpretation of smells and sounds.

1.3.4 The Occipital Lobe

The *occipital lobe* is located in the back portion of the brain behind the parietal and temporal lobes, and is primarily responsible for processing visual information. The occipital lobe contains the brain's visual processing system: it processes images from our eyes and links that information with images stored in memory. The occipital lobe, the smallest of the four lobes, is located near the posterior region of the cerebral cortex, near the back of the skull. It is the primary visual processing center of the brain; other functions include[9,10]

- visual-spatial processing
- movement and color recognition.

1.4 ELECTROENCEPHALOGRAPHY

Electroencephalography (EEG) is a non-invasive brain-imaging method that records the brain's electrical activity at the surface of the scalp. EEG was first used in 1929 by Hans Berger, who recorded brain activity beneath the closed skull and reported changes during different states. In 1957 Gray Walter was the first person to record the brain with electrodes, and showed that brain rhythms changed according to different mental tasks.

EEG equipment usually comes in the form of a cap or headset that has several electrodes or sensors which are designed to fix to the surface of the head.[11] An EEG device records electrical signals from the brain, specifically postsynaptic potentials of neurons, through electrodes attached either to the subject's scalp, the subdural (ie, beneath the dura matter—the outermost, toughest, and most fibrous of three membranes covering and protecting the brain and spinal cord), or even the cortex itself (these latter two cases are relatively rare). EEGs are based upon the theory of volume conduction of ionic current through nonempty extracellular space. The recording is obtained by placing electrodes on the scalp, usually after some abrasion and with a conductive gel to create a better contact. The measured EEG activity is the sum of all the synchronous activity of all the neurons in the area below the electrode that have the same approximate vertical orientation to the scalp. Fig. 1.4A and B shows the activity in the brain after electrodes are placed on the scalp using the illustrated EEG cap.

An EEG is used to diagnose certain brain disorders. The measurements given by an EEG are used to provide information about disorders such as:

- seizure disorders, including epilepsy
- head injury
- encephalitis, or inflammation of the brain
- brain tumor
- encephalopathy, or brain dysfunction resulting from various causes
- memory problems
- stroke
- sleep disorders.[12,13]

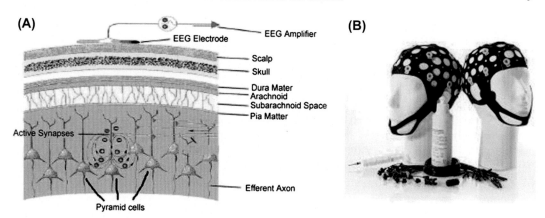

FIGURE 1.4 (A) Activity in brain after placing the electrodes; (B) EEG cap.

1.5 HUMAN AUDITORY SYSTEM

To plan a speech-based interface system, it is significant to comprehend the working of the human auditory system. At the linguistic level of communication, an idea is first formed in the mind of the speaker, and then produced in the form of speech. The idea is transformed into words, phrases, and sentences according to the grammatical rules of the language. At the physiological point of communication, the brain creates electric signals that travel along the motor nerves. These electric signals activate muscles in the vocal tract and vocal cords. This vocal tract and vocal cord movement results in pressure changes within the vocal tract and in particular at the lips, initiating sound waves that propagate into space. Finally, at the linguistic level of the listener, the brain performs speech recognition and understanding.[14–16] Besides interactive command and control signals, it is efficient in expressing emotions. This effectiveness can be examined to build robust emotion recognition systems.

1.5.1 Speech Production Mechanism

Human speech is brought out by complex interactions between the diaphragm, lungs, pharynx, mouth, and nasal cavity. The procedures which control speech production are phonation, resonation, and articulation. Phonation is the process of converting air pressure into sound via the vocal folds, or vocal cords. Resonation is the process by which certain frequencies are emphasized by resonances in the vocal tract. Articulation is the procedure of altering the vocal tract resonances to produce distinguishable sounds.

Air enters the lungs via the normal breathing mechanism. As air is released from the lungs through the trachea, the tensed vocal cords within the larynx are made to oscillate by the air stream. The air-flow is chopped into quasiperiodic pulses, which are modulated in frequency by passing through the pharynx, mouth cavity, and nasal cavity. Depending on the status of various articulators, different sounds are made. The lungs and associated muscles act as the source of air for exciting the vocal mechanism. The muscle force pushes air out of the lungs through the bronchi and trachea.[17]

All the sounds generated when we speak are the result of muscles contracting. The muscles in the chest that we use for breathing produce the flow of air that is needed for almost all speech sounds; muscles in the larynx produce many different modifications in the flow of air from the chest to the mouth. After going through the larynx, the air travels through what we call the vocal tract, which terminates at the mouth and nostrils. Here the air from the lungs escapes into the atmosphere. We have a large and complex set of muscles that can produce changes in the shape of the vocal tract, and to learn how the sounds of speech are produced it is necessary to become familiar with the different parts of the vocal tract. These different parts are called articulators, and the study of them is called articulatory phonetics.

The organs involved in the production of speech are depicted in Fig. 1.5. It represents the human head, seen from the side, displayed as though it had been cut in half.

1. The pharynx is a tube which begins just above the larynx. It is nearly 7 cm long in women and about 8 cm in men, and at its top end is divided into two, one part being the back of the oral cavity and the other being the beginning of the path through the nasal cavity.
2. The velum or soft palate is seen in the diagram in a position that allows air to pass through the nose and mouth. The other important thing about the velum is that it is one of the articulators that can be touched by the tongue.
3. The hard palate is often named the "roof of the oral cavity."

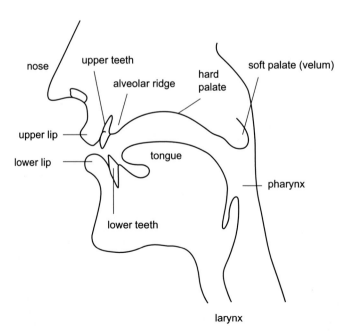

FIGURE 1.5   The articulators.

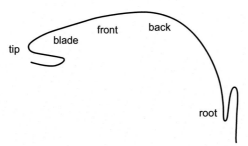

FIGURE 1.6   Subdivisions of the tongue.

4. The alveolar ridge is between the top front teeth and the hard palate. Its surface is very much more grating than it feels, and is covered with short ridges. Sounds made with the tongue touching here (such as *t* and *d*) are called alveolar.

5. The tongue is a very important articulator, and can be moved into many different places and shapes. It is usual to divide the tongue into parts, though there are no clear dividing lines within the tongue. Fig. 1.6 shows the tongue on a larger scale: tip, blade, front, back, and root.

6. The tongue is in touch with the upper side teeth for many speech sounds. Sounds made with the tongue touching the front teeth are called dental.

7. The lips are important in speech. They can be pressed together (when we produce the sounds *p*, *b*), brought into contact with the teeth (as in *f*, *v*), or rounded to produce the lip shape for vowels like *uù*. Sounds in which the lips are in contact with each other are called bilabial, while those with lip-to-teeth contact are called labiodentals.

From a signal-oriented point of view, the production of speech is widely described as a two-level process. In the first stage the sound is initiated, and in the second phase it is filtered along the second level. This distinction between phases has its source in the source-filter model of speech production. Fig. 1.7 shows a source signal produced at the glottal level.[18]

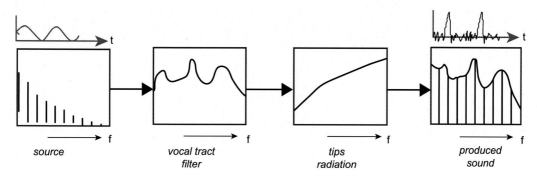

FIGURE 1.7   Source signal produced at the glottal level.

The basic premise of the model is that a source signal produced at the glottal level is linearly filtered through the vocal tract. The resulting sound is given off to the surrounding air through radiation loading (lips). The model assumes that source and filter are independent of each other. Although recent findings indicate more or less interaction between the vocal tract and a glottal source, Fant's theory[19] of language production is still used as a framework for the description of the human voice, particularly as far as the articulation of vowels is concerned.

From a linguistic phonetic point of view, the production of speech is regarded as a superposition of initiation, phonation, articulation, and prosodic organization processes. Fig. 1.8 shows the mechanisms involved in the production of speech sounds: lungs, glottis, and vocal tract.[20]

Speech is produced as a sequence of sounds. The articulators such as jaw, tongue, velum, lips, and mouth and their shapes, sizes, and positions change over time to produce sounds. In the physiological aspects we can split up the speech production process into three different levels.

1. Conceptualization.
2. Formulation.
3. Articulation.

Fig. 1.9 shows the flow of speech production. Speech actually starts from our brain as a thought process, when it can be considered as a preverbal message. This procedure is known

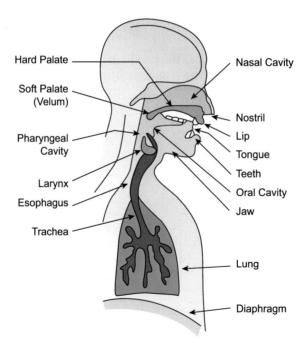

FIGURE 1.8   Speech production mechanisms.

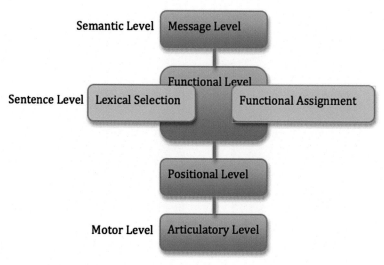

FIGURE 1.9   Flowchart for speech production.

as conceptualization. The second stage of the speech production process is speech formulation, when our thought (preverbal message) is converted into linguistic form. This stage is subdivided into two parts.

1. Lexicalization: here our thought will be converted into appropriate words.
2. Syntactic planning: here, the appropriate words will be arranged in the right (syntactically correct) way.

The voice is the terminal phase of speech output, when sounds will be produced to convey the message.[21]

1.6   SPEECH PROCESSING

Speech is the main modality of communication among human beings, and the most natural and effective way of exchanging information between humans. Speech processing is a discipline of computer science that deals with designing computer systems that recognize spoken words. The technology permits a data processor to identify the words that a person speaks into a microphone or phone. Automatic speech recognition is defined as the process of converting a speech signal to a sequence of words by means of an algorithm implemented by computer program,[22,23] and is one of the fastest developing fields in the framework of speech science and engineering.

The goal of speech processing is to develop techniques and real-time automatic speech understanding systems. The motivation is to modernize computer systems so they behave as a reliever for a human expert.

The study of speech ranges from technological curiosity about the mechanisms of realization of human speech capabilities to work on automating simple tasks which require

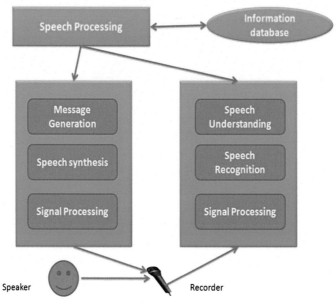

FIGURE 1.10   Basic architecture of a speech processing system.

human—machine interaction. The concept of machines being able to interact with people in natural frames is very attractive. Few commercial products of varying capabilities are already available, where they are operated by issuing spoken commands to get corresponding relevant response.

Automatic speech processing is a technology which digitizes spoken words, identifies individual sounds (phonemes), and use mathematical models to select discrete words or phrases. This speech processing is a particular example of pattern recognition. The basic architecture of automatic speech processing implementation is depicted in Fig. 1.10.

To generalize the use of such systems in different man—machine interaction contexts, a predictive model of performance needs to be obtained as a function of different identified relevant factors. In speech processing, the human auditory system plays a significant part.

Likewise, the accent, speaking style, age group, and mother tongue are speech-intrinsic variations in which emotional state is grounded to influence the language spectrum significantly. It is recognized that mood change in a speaker has a considerable impact on the features extracted from his/her speech, hence directly affecting the basis of all speech recognition systems. Studies on speakers' emotions are a fairly recent and emerging area. Interesting studies have been carried out to classify a "stressed" or "frustrated" speech signal into its correct emotion category.[24—27]

1.6.1 Speech Emotion Recognition

Automatic emotion recognition from speech signals has become a major research subject in the area of human—computer interaction in recent times due to its many potential applications. It is being used in a number of emerging areas, such as humanoid robots, the car industry, call centers, mobile communication, computer tutorial applications, etc.

Many features have been proposed for speech-based emotion recognition, and a majority of them are frame based or statistics estimated from frame-based features. Temporal information is typically modeled on a per utterance basis, with either functional or frame-based features or a suitable back-end.

Speech is a key communication modality for humans to encode emotion. Emotional speech production, acoustic feature extraction for emotion analysis, and the design of a speech-based emotion recognizer are the challenging domains in the current research era.

Emotion labeling (or annotation) typically offers a ground truth for training and evaluating emotion recognition systems. The specific selection of representations (descriptors) used for computing depends on the theoretical underpinnings and the application goal. In addition to traditionally used categorical (happy, angry, sad, and indifferent) and dimensional (arousal, valence, and dominance) labels, researchers have made advances in computationally integrating behavior described in the depiction of emotion.

Most studies of emotional speech have focused on the acoustic characteristics of the resulting speech signal level, such as the underlying prosodic variation, spectral shape, and voice quality change, across various timescales, rather than considering the underlying production mechanisms directly. To understand the complex acoustic structure and further the human communication process that involves information encoding and decoding, a deeper understanding of orchestrated articulator activity is needed.[28]

1.7 ORGANIZATION OF THE BOOK

The book aims at emotion recognition through two major sources of emotion: the brain where emotions are generated, and the speech which communicates them. The presentation of brain physiology is important in understanding the brain signals, which are represented as brain waves or rhythms. Study of human auditory system helps us to understand speech generation and processing. Emotions can be observed through the acoustic parameters of speech. As emotion cannot be recognized through a single cue, multiple cues can help in developing robust emotion recognition systems.

Chapter "Technological Basics of EEG Recording and Operation of Apparatus" is concerned with the technological basics of EEG recording and operation of apparatus. The chapter gives a basic introduction to EEG, brain waves, and the functioning of a typical EEG machine. It also illustrates the 10/20 placement system of electrodes through which brain signals are acquired. It presents a detailed description of an RMS EEG machine as an example, with its available utilities and operation. It also describes a computerized speech laboratory and speech acquisition and analysis equipment, along with its operation for speech processing.

Chapter "Technical Aspects of Brain Rhythms and Speech Parameters" describes technical aspects of brain rhythms and speech parameters. It introduces details of all five types of brain rhythms (ie, gamma, alpha, beta, theta, and delta). This chapter presents the important parameters for speech analysis considering emotions. Parameters related to prosody signal measures, spectral characteristics, and voice quality measures are explained, followed by the techniques of preprocessing, feature extraction, and feature classification.

Chapter "Time and Frequency Analysis" illustrates the details of time domain and frequency domain techniques.

Chapter "Emotion Recognition" introduces emotion recognition with modalities researched. Features used in different modalities for six basic emotions (happiness, sadness, anger, fear, disgust, and surprise) are explained. The face, speech, gesture, text, and EEG signals are the modalities described, along with the databases available for research.

Chapter "Multimodal Emotion Recognition" gives details about multimodal emotion recognition systems. It reviews different modalities used to recognize emotion, and focuses on the need for multimodal concept. A summary of online available databases for multimodal systems is presented. Advantages and challenges with such systems, models of emotions, and earlier research are also discussed.

Chapter "Proposed EEG—Speech Based Emotion Recognition System: A Case Study" presents details of a real-world case study for a multimodal emotion recognition system. It begins with the Emotional Intelligence Inventory used for the selection of volunteers. It explores the database creation, correlation, and experimentation done with EEG images and speech signals for recognition using linear discriminate analysis for two basic emotions, happiness and sadness.

Chapter "BCI and Its Applications" introduces how brain—computer interfacing works, and describes the potential application of brain—computer interfacing such as P300, home automation, lie detector brain fingerprinting, and mood assessment.

1.8 CONCLUSION

Communication through emotions is a common phenomenon in human beings, but it is still in its infancy in digital technology. For digital representation, one needs to understand quantifications of emotions as well as signals associated with generation of these emotions. Emotions can be shown in multiple ways, such as speech, hand gestures, facial expressions, etc., but all are produced and controlled by the brain. As different emotions are generated by different regions of the brain, it is important to understand the functioning of these regions. Similarly, emotions generated by speech are dependent on human auditory systems. This chapter gives introductory descriptions of these three aspects—emotions, brain, and speech—of which an understanding is needed to develop emotion-based digital technology.

References

1. Rached TS, Perkusich A. *Emotion Recognition Based on Brain-Computer Interface Systems, Brain-Computer Interface Systems — Recent Progress and Future.* InTech; 2013. http://dx.doi.org/10.5772/56227. ISBN 978-953-51-1134-4.
2. *Structure of Emotions.* http://www.britannica.com/topic/emotion/The-structure-of-emotions.
3. Plutchik R. https://en.wikipedia.org/wiki/Robert_Plutchik.
4. Mangal SK. *An Introduction to Psychology.* Sterling Publishers Private Ltd; 2013.
5. *Brain Structures and Their Functions.* http://serendip.brynmawr.edu/bb/kinser/Structure1.html.
6. Ekman P. Chapter 3: basic emotions. In: Dalgleish T, Power M, eds. *Handbook of Cognition and Emotion.* Sussex, U.K.: John Wiley & Sons, Ltd; 1999.
7. Socrates. *Chapter 1: Know Yourself—Lesson 4: Brain Structure and Function, Unit 3: Foundations for Success.*
8. *Emotional Lateralization.* https://en.wikipedia.org/wiki/Emotional_lateralization.

9. Fralich T, LCPC. *Emotions, Mindfulness and the Pathways of the Brain.*
10. *The Anatomy of the Brain.* http://psychology.about.com/od/biopsychology/ss/brainstructure_2.htm#step-heading.
11. *Electroencephalography.* http://en.wikipedia.org/wiki/Electroencephalography.
12. Nunez PL. *Neocortical Dynamics and Human EEG Rhythms.* New York: Oxford University Press; 1995.
13. *Fundamentals of Electroencephalogram.* www.eelab.usyd.edu.au/ELEC3801/notes/Electroencephalogram.htm.
14. Rabiner L, Juang BH. *Fundamentals of Speech Approach.* Prentice Hall PTR; 1993.
15. Quatieri TF. *Discrete-Time Speech Signal Processing: Principles and Practice.* Pearson Education, Inc.; 2002.
16. Rabiner LR. *Speech Recognition by Machine.* CRC Press LLC; 2000.
17. Rabiner L, Juang BH, Yegnanarayana B. *Fundamentals of Speech Recognition.* Pearson; 1993. ISBN 978-81-775-8560-5.
18. *Articulator System.* http://www.personal.rdg.ac.uk/~llsroach/phon2/artic-basics.htm.
19. *Fant's Theory.* https://en.wikipedia.org/wiki/Gunnar_Fant.
20. *Source Signal Production.* http://www2.ims.uni-stuttgart.de/EGG/page4.htm.
21. *Speech Production Mechanism.* http://www.academia.edu/3052872/Speech_Production_mechanism.
22. Gaikwad S, Gawali B, Yannawar P. A review on speech recognition technique. *Int J Comput Appl.* November 2010;10(3). ISSN:0975-8887.
23. Picheny M. Large vocabulary speech recognition. *Computer.* 2002;35(4):42–50.
24. Roux JC, Botha EC, Du Preez JA. Developing a multilingual telephone based information system in African languages. In: *Proceedings of the Second International Language Resources and Evaluation Conference.* vol. 2. Athens, Greece: ELRA; 2000:975–980.
25. Robertson J, Wong YT, Chung C, Kim DK. Automatic speech recognition for generalized time based media retrieval and indexing. In: *Proceedings of the Sixth ACM International Conference on Multimedia.* Bristol, England; 1998:241–246.
26. *Embedded Speech Solutions.* Retrieved January 25, 2013: http://www.speechworks.com/.
27. Kandasamy S. Speech recognition systems. *SURPRISE J.* 1995;1(1).
28. Ayadi ME, Kamel MS, Karray F. Survey on speech emotion recognition: features, classification schemes, and databases. *Pattern Recognit.* March 2011;44(3):572–587.

Technological Basics of EEG Recording and Operation of Apparatus

Introduction to EEG- and Speech-Based Emotion Recognition
http://dx.doi.org/10.1016/B978-0-12-804490-2.00002-6

19

2.1 INTRODUCTION TO ELECTROENCEPHALOGRAPHY

Electroencephalography (EEG), a noninvasive medical imaging technique, is defined as an electrical activity recorded from the surface of the scalp with the help of metal electrodes and a conducting medium. For clinical neurophysiology and neurology, EEG has been found to be very useful. An electroencephalogram (also abbreviated as EEG) measured directly from the cortical surface is called an electrocardiogram, while when using depth probes it is called an electrogram. A local current is generated when neurons in the brain are activated during synaptic excitations of the dendrites, and is measured as EEG. Differences of electrical potentials are caused by summed postsynaptic graded potentials from pyramidal cells that create electrical dipoles between soma (body of neuron) and apical dendrites (neural branches).[1]

Electroencephalographic reading is a completely safe procedure that can be conducted repeatedly on patients, normal adults, and children without any risk or limitation. The local current flow is caused by active neurons consisting of Na^+, K^+, Ca^{++}, and Cl^- ions that are expelled through channels in neuron membranes in the direction governed by membrane potential.[2] The recordable electrical activity is created on the head surface. Between electrode and neuronal layers the current penetrates through skin, skull, and several other layers. The signals detected through electrodes are weak, so they are amplified, digitized, and stored to computer memory.[3] EEG is a useful medical tool as it has the ability to record both normal and abnormal electrical activity of the brain.[4]

The highest influence on EEG comes from electrical activity of the cerebral cortex, due to its surface position.[5,6]

During its more than 100-year history, EEG has made massive progress. Berger laid the foundations for many of its present applications, and also first used the word electroencephalogram for describing brain electric potentials in humans. He found that brain activity changes in a consistent and recognizable way when the general status of the subject changes, as from relaxation to alertness. Later, in 1934, Adrian and Matthews published a paper verifying the concept of "human brain waves" and identified regular oscillations around 10–12 Hz, which they termed "alpha rhythm."[7]

2.1.1 Brain Waves

Brain waves are oscillating electrical voltages in the brain measuring just a few millionths of a volt. There are five widely recognized brain waves, and the main frequencies of human EEG waves are listed in Table 2.1 along with their characteristics.

Brain wave samples for different waveforms are shown in Fig. 2.1.

Various regions of the brain do not emit the same brain wave frequency simultaneously. An EEG signal between electrodes placed on the scalp consists of many waves with different characteristics. The large amount of data received from even one single EEG recording makes interpretation difficult. The brain wave patterns are unique for every individual.[8]

TABLE 2.1   Characteristics of the Five Basic Brain Waves

Frequency band	Frequency	Brain states
Gamma (γ)	>35 Hz	Concentration
Beta (β)	12–35 Hz	Anxiety dominant, active, external attention, relaxed
Alpha (α)	8–12 Hz	Very relaxed, passive attention
Theta (θ)	4–8 Hz	Deeply relaxed, inward focused
Delta (δ)	0.5–4 Hz	Sleep

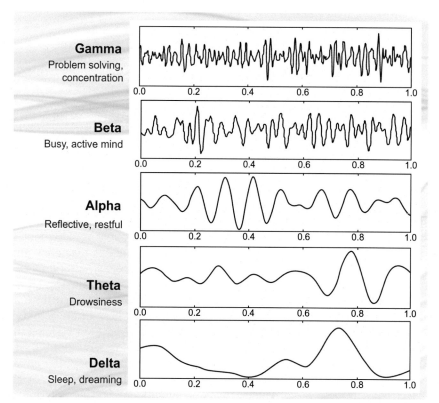

FIGURE 2.1   Brain wave samples with dominant frequencies belonging to beta, alpha, theta, and delta bands and gamma waves.

2.1.2 Applications of EEG

EEG has applications in various domains. Some applications[9] in humans and animals can be listed as follows.

1. Monitor alertness, coma, and brain death.
2. Locate areas of damage following head injury, stroke, tumor, etc.
3. Test afferent pathways.
4. Monitor cognitive engagement.
5. Produce biofeedback situations, alpha, etc.
6. Control anesthesia depth.
7. Investigate epilepsy and locate seizure origin.
8. Test epilepsy drug effects.
9. Assist in experimental cortical excision of epileptic focus.
10. Monitor human and animal brain development.
11. Test drugs for convulsive effects.
12. Investigate sleep disorder and physiology.

2.2 MODERN EEG EQUIPMENT

With the advent of digital technology, EEG systems are being developed in various directions. Digital systems have advantages which make them capable of special applications. Signal storage, retrieval, numeric processing, and novel display are among the capabilities of digital systems. The companies developing EEG machines differentiate themselves based on features, performance, and cost.

Postacquisition tools such as spectral arrays are available now with EEG applications from a variety of suppliers. They run on laptop computers that are cheaper, faster, and more powerful than those available to the earlier investigators. The development of digital EEG for routine recording has produced a relatively cheap and robust replacement for EEGs that used paper technology. Recordings are carried out on digital machines and can be viewed with different montages, filter settings, and display speeds; additional procedures such as voltage mapping or frequency analysis can also be carried out. Digital media can be used to store recordings, thus EEGs are archived. EEGs can be accessed from anywhere in the world through simple and cheap file transfer protocols.[10] Brain activity may be recorded by means of wired or wireless EEG systems. With wired EEG systems the subject must remain constrained in one location, so recently developers have optimized wireless EEG systems that facilitate mobile recordings of the brain activity. These offer an advantage compared to wired systems because the person is less restricted in movement range and types. The electronics are also much smaller than in conventional devices, and do not require a cable to transmit the data from the EEG cap to the computer. The following subsections present the merits and demerits of wired and wireless EEG systems.

2.2.1 Wired EEG Systems

2.2.1.1 *Merits*

- The latest digital design techniques take advantage of years of expertise in amplifier design and manufacturing. Easily identifiable electrode input using the international 10–20 placement layout is helpful in placing the electrodes on the scalp.
- The user interface with liquid crystal display allows information such as electrode impedance checking, amplifier calibration, photic stimulator control, and connection status to be observed.
- More than 72 h of EEG data can be acquired, which can be useful for studying seizures and spike detection.
- In the early days of brain computer interfacing (BCI) research, cursor control and speller applications were developed, mainly targeted at helping disabled people.[11]

2.2.1.2 *Demerits*

- It is time-consuming: setting up an EEG can take 25–45 min.
- Loose, spread-out wires result in an antenna effect and can cause electrical artifacts and spurious results.
- Many conventional BCI systems are wired. With just three electrodes positioned at the occipital lobe, the acquisition part of wired BCI systems generally comes with bulky and heavy amplifiers and preprocessing units.
- Wires of electrodes restrict the mobility of the subject.
- Connection wiring is usually complicated, with a large number of cables between the electrodes and the acquisition machine.[12]

2.2.2 Wireless EEG Systems

2.2.2.1 *Merits*

- A wireless BCI system eliminates the wire connection with the use of a wireless transmission unit such as Bluetooth and Zigbee modules.
- The wireless mode makes the system portable.
- Wearing during acquisition is easy, so the postures and movements of users are comfortable. These desirable changes in wireless BCI systems take the technique beyond laboratory experiments and into everyday-life applications.
- Recently, with growing interest, wireless BCI systems have been applied in entertainment. For example, the Emotiv and Neurosky companies have released wireless BCI headsets for entertainment uses such as brain gaming and mind monitoring.
- International research groups have applied wireless BCI systems in interesting new applications such as home automation systems based on monitoring human physiological states, cellular phone dialing, and drowsiness detection for drivers.

2.2.2.2 Demerits

- The features are limited, as it can interpret only simple messages from user intentions.
- In wireless systems many features of the EEG signals, such as cognitive states and event-related potentials (ERPs), can be easily affected by external noises.
- Wireless systems provide less accuracy.[13]

2.2.3 Evoked Potentials

An **evoked potential** or **evoked response** is an electrical potential recorded from the nervous system of a human or animal following presentation of a stimulus, as distinct from spontaneous potentials as detected by EEG, electromyography (EMG), or other electrophysiological recording methods. Evoked potentials ERPs are significant voltage fluctuations resulting from evoked neural activity. The technique is best suited to studying the aspects of cognitive processes in both normal and abnormal states.

Evoked potential amplitudes tend to be low. Signal averaging is applied to resolve these low-amplitude potentials running in the background of ongoing EEG and other biological signals. The signal is time-locked to the stimulus and most of the noise occurs randomly, allowing the noise to be averaged out by averaging repeated responses.[9]

2.3 THE EEG 10/20 ELECTRODES PLACEMENT SYSTEM

Encephalographic measurements employ a recording system comprising:

- electrodes with conductive media
- amplifiers with filters
- analog-to-digital (A/D) converter
- recording device

The standard placement is that recommended by the American EEG Society. The standard numbering system places odd-numbered electrodes on the left of the scalp and even-numbered electrodes on the right side of the scalp. The numbers 10 and 20 refer to distances between adjacent electrodes placed at either 10% or 20% distance on the skull. Electrode locations are determined by dividing these perimeters into 10% and 20% intervals. F describes frontal regions, C describes the central region, P is for the parietal region, and T is for temporal. Z refers to electrodes placed on the midline. The anterior is represented by symbol A. For the corporal landmarks some fundamental positions are taken in consideration:

1. nasion
2. inion
3. preauricular point

In this system 21 electrodes are located on the surface of the scalp, and gather EEG signals produced by electrical activity in the brain. Fig. 2.2 shows the labeled 10/20 international electrode placement system.

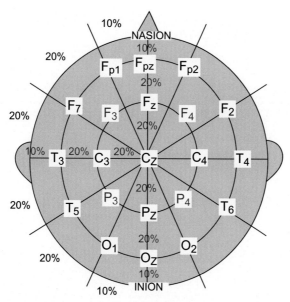

FIGURE 2.2   The 10/20 international electrode placement system.

When recording a more detailed EEG, extra electrodes are added to the spaces in between the existing 10/20 system. This new electrode naming system is more complicated, giving rise to the modified combinatorial nomenclature (MCN). The MCN system uses 1, 3, 5, 7, and 9 for the left hemisphere, representing 10%, 20%, 30%, 40%, and 50% of the inion-to-nasion distance respectively; while 2, 4, 6, 8, and 10 are used for the right hemisphere. The introduction of extra letters allows the naming of extra electrode sites.

Scalp recordings of neuronal activity in the brain, identified as the EEG, allow measurement of potential changes over time in basic electric circuit conducting between the signal (active) electrode and the reference electrode.[16] An extra third electrode, called the ground electrode, is needed to get differential voltage by subtracting the same voltages shown at active and reference points. The minimal configuration for monochannel EEG measurement consists of one active electrode, one (or two specially linked together) reference electrode and one ground electrode. Multichannel configurations can comprise up to 128 or 256 active electrodes.

With modern instrumentation, the choice of a ground electrode plays no significant role in the measurement.[14] A forehead (Fpz) or ear location is preferred,[15] but sometimes a wrist or leg is used. The channels are composed of the combination of all electrodes along with reference and ground electrodes. The general configuration is called a montage.

Electrodes read the signal from the head surface, amplifiers bring the microvolt signals into the range where they can be digitalized accurately, the converter changes signals from analog to digital form, and a computer (or other relevant device) stores and displays acquired data. A set of this equipment is shown in Fig. 2.3.

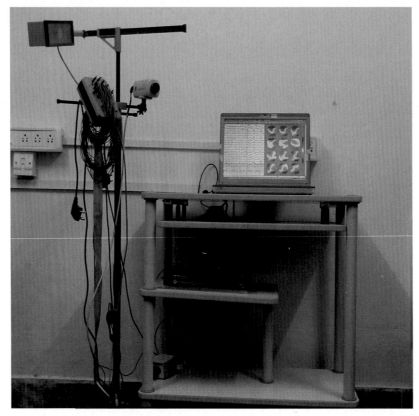

FIGURE 2.3   Equipment for EEG recording.

The EEG recording electrodes and their proper function are critical for acquiring appropriate high-quality data for interpretation. Electrodes are of different types:

- disposable (gel-less and pregelled types)
- reusable disc electrodes (gold, silver, stainless steel, or tin)
- headbands and electrode caps
- saline-based electrodes
- needle electrodes

Commonly used scalp electrodes consist of Ag–AgCl disks, 1–3 mm in diameter, with long flexible leads that can be plugged into an amplifier.[7] AgCl electrodes can accurately record very slow changes in potential.[9] Needle electrodes are used for long recordings and are invasively inserted under the scalp.

For recording it is advised to have clean skin free of oil or any other stickiness. With disposable and disc electrodes, abrasive paste is used for slight skin abrasion. With cap systems, an abutting needle is used for skin scraping, which can cause irritation, pain, and infection.

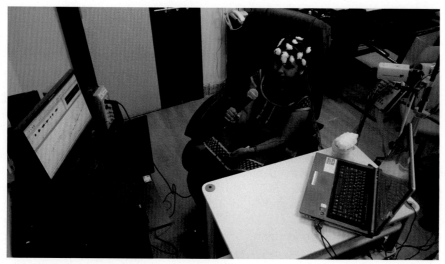

FIGURE 2.4   Acquisition setup for EEG and CSL speech signals.

If silver—silver chloride electrodes are used, the space between the electrode and the skin is filled with conductive paste to help adhesion. With cap systems there is a small hole to inject conductive jelly. Conductive paste and conductive jelly serve as media to ensure lowering of contact impedance at the electrode—skin interface (Fig. 2.4).

Different brain areas are related to different functions of the brain. Each scalp electrode is located near a particular brain center, for example:

- F7 is located near centers for rational activities
- Fz is near intentional and motivational centers
- F8 is close to sources of emotional impulses
- the cortex around C3, C4, and Cz deals with sensory and motor functions
- P3, P4, and Pz locations contribute to activity of perception and differentiation
- near T3 and T4 emotional processors are located
- T5 and T6 are near certain memory functions
- primary visual areas can be found below points O1 and O2

However, the scalp electrodes may not reflect the particular areas of the cortex, as the exact location of the active sources is still a problem due to limitations caused by the nonhomogeneous properties of the skull, different orientation of the cortex sources, coherence between the sources, etc.[4]

Several different recording reference electrode placements are mentioned in the literature. Physical references can be chosen as:

- vertex (Cz)
- linked ears
- linked mastoids
- ipsilateral ear
- contralateral ear

- C7 reference
- bipolar references
- tip of the nose

Reference-free techniques are represented by common average reference, weighted average reference, and source derivation.

2.4 EEG ACQUISITION TOOL

There are many EEG machines available: Neuroscan, WinEEG Advanced EEG, MAXIMUS 24/32*, and many more. The RMS EEG 32-channel 19-electrodes machine is described as an example of the equipment.[17] RMS stands for Recorders and Medicare System, a company manufacturing equipment such as EEG, EMG, electrocardiogram (ECG), polysomnography (PSG), transcranial Doppler, and many other machines.[18] The RMS EEG 32-channel 19-electrodes machine, which includes an AC impedance check, gives simultaneous acquisition of raw data and is used for experimental purposes. Techniques and facilities available include color brain mapping, signal analysis, time/frequency operations, etc. The machine has a panel for connection of wired metal-plated electrodes, which are placed on the scalp of the subject, and includes a camera which is used to capture the movements of the subject (Fig. 2.5). It also includes two software programs: "Acquire" and "Analysis."

2.4.1 EEG Acquire Software

The Acquire software is used to record (acquire) data from the scalp of the subject. The software uses various icons (Fig. 2.6).

- **File New Info** prior to the experiment, data on the subject is compiled in "File-new patient," including the patient/subject's name, doctor's name, age, gender, and some other details. An example is shown in Fig. 2.7.
- **File-PtInfo** provides existing information on the subject.
- **Acquisition-Cal** displays the calibration of individual channels as per **cal rate** (in Hz) and **cal level** (in μV).
- **Acquisition-EEG** shows the incoming EEG data in the form of signals.
- **Acquisition-Impedance Check** shows the impedance of each electrode (Fig. 2.8). **Opn** stands for an open electrode, ie, not connected or not connected properly. The impedance may be set to an acceptable limit. When the impedance of electrodes exceeds this limit the electrode is set to be red, otherwise it turns green. The default limit of impedance is generally set as 20 KOhms. The impedance related to each experiment for every subject can be saved.
- **Acquisition-StartEEG** starts acquisition of the EEG waveforms.
- **Acquisition-Stop** stops the acquisition.
- **Acquisition-Record** starts recording the EEG. During recording autoprotocol or manual mode can be used to mark events in time. The facility to mark comments is also available.

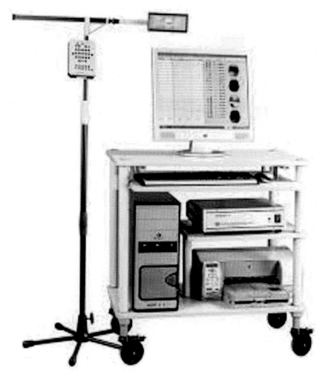

FIGURE 2.5   The RMS EEG 32-channel machine.

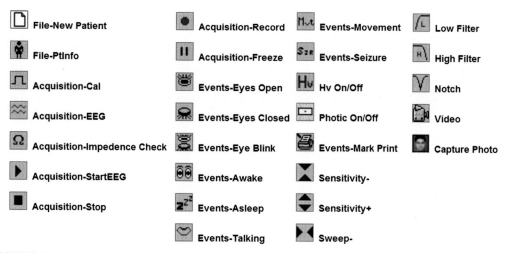

FIGURE 2.6   Icons in toolbar of Acquire software for EEG.

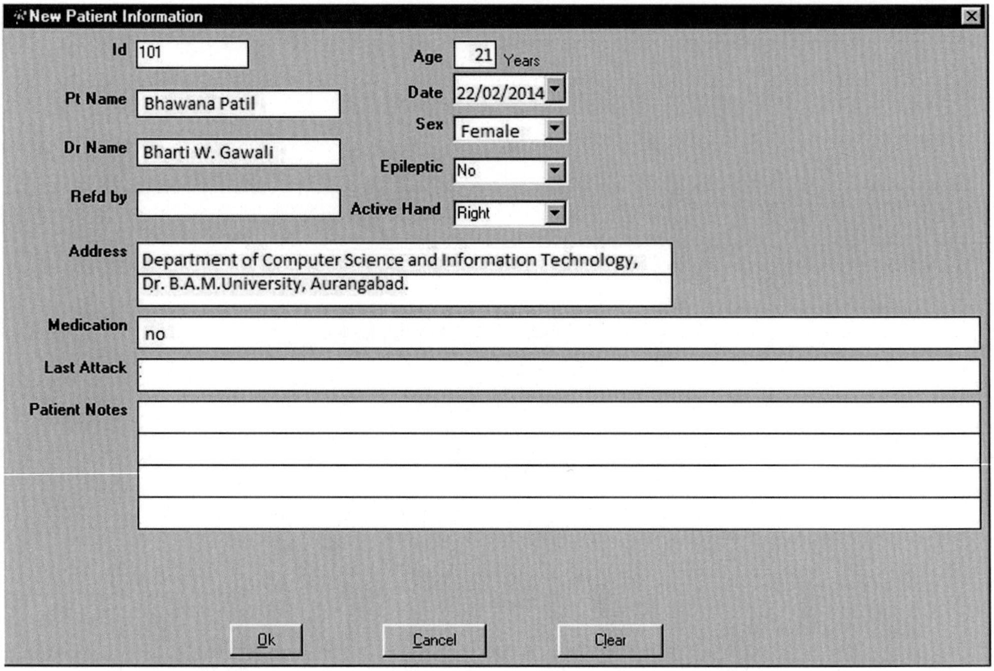

FIGURE 2.7   New patient information for acquiring EEG.

- **Acquisition-Freeze** is used to freeze the signals while recording.
  This machine provides 14 predefined events, and users can select an event as and when required. Some examples of events are
  - eyes open
  - eyes closed
  - eyes blink
  - awake
  - asleep
  - talking
  - movement
  - seizure
- **HV (hyperventilate)** will toggle to put a mark for HV on or off at the desired time during recording.
- **Photic** mode can be set manually or even automatically. The value set should be between 5 and 15 s.
- **Sensitivity** changes the sensitivity. Options are 1, 2, 3, 5, 7.5, 10, 15, 20, 30, 50, 75, 100, 150, 200, 300, 500, 750, and 1000 µV/mm. The sensitivity can be increased or decreased.
- **Sweep** changes the sweep. Options are 7.5, 15, 30, and 60 mm/s.
- **Low Filter** changes the value of the lower filter. Options are DC, 0.1, 0.3, 0.5, 1.0, 3.0, and 5.0.

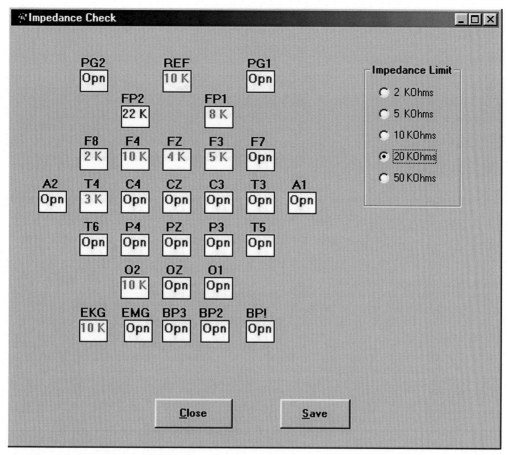

FIGURE 2.8   Acquisition-impedance check of a patient for EEG.

- **High Filter** changes the value of the high filter. Options are 15, 35, 70, and also user defined in Hz.
- **Notch** changes the value of the notch. Options are none, 50, and 60 Hz.
- **Video** can be used to capture the movements of the patient or subject.
- **Capture Photo** is used to take a photo of the patient or subject for the record.[18]

2.4.2 EEG Analysis Software

The Analysis software is used to analyze the subject data gained using the Acquire software; its various icons are shown in Fig. 2.9.

- **File-Ptinfo** opens the patient information windows and gives details of the patient.
- **File-Open** gives a list of patients and opens the existing **.eeg file**.
- **File-Print** displays the window to print the page.

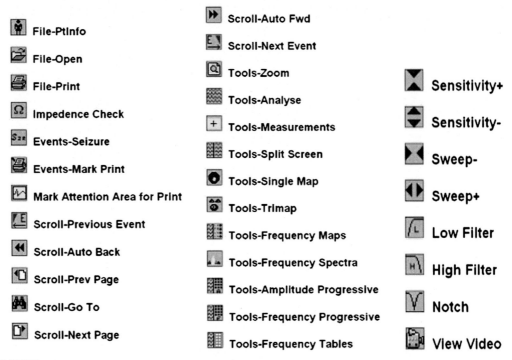

FIGURE 2.9   Icons in toolbar of Analysis software for EEG.

- **Events-Seizure** enables the user to select the desired event.
- **Events-Mark Print** prints the event marked while acquiring the EEG.
- **Scroll-Previous Event** scrolls the cursor to move to the previous event.
- **Scroll-Prev Page** moves the cursor to the previous page.
- **Scroll-Next Page** moves the cursor to the next page.
- **Scroll-Go To** enables the user to go to the set location.
- **Scroll-Auto Fwd** scrolls the page in auto-forward form.
- **Tools-Single Map**: Fig. 2.10 shows the instance of EEG signals viewed in an amplitude map. The values of that instance are seen against the name of each electrode.
- **Tools-Trimap**: Fig. 2.11 presents the instance of EEG signals viewed in an amplitude map. The left, right, and top views can be seen. The values of that instance are seen against the name of each electrode.
- **Tools-Frequency Maps**: Fig. 2.12 shows the frequency map, where the yellow bar of EEG trace represents 2 s of selected EEG for frequency analysis. The right side shows power spectra in δ, θ, α and β bands, PPF (peak power frequency), and the contribution of each band to the total power for each electrode. Each band is represented by a different color:

    $\delta = 0-4$ Hz, color is red

    $\theta = 4-8$ Hz, color is yellow

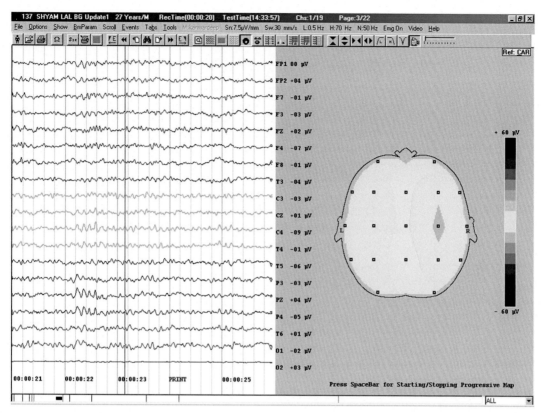

FIGURE 2.10   EEG single map.

$\alpha = 8-12$ Hz, color is green

$\beta = 12-16$ Hz, color is blue

The PPF color represents the band in which this peak occurs. The four maps on the right are frequency maps for four frequency bands. The sensitivity of power spectra and maps can be changed from the BmParam menu by selecting FreqMapSen.

- **Tools-Frequency Spectra**: Fig. 2.13 shows the frequency spectra. The yellow bar of EEG trace represents 2 s of EEG selected for frequency spectra. The right side shows power spectra for all 21 electrodes. It also shows
  - **PPF**, ie, the frequency at which the peak power occurs)
  - **SEF** (spectral edge frequency), ie, the frequency below which lies the 95% power of the spectra)
  - **MPF** (median power frequency), ie, where 50% of power is below and 50% is above this frequency, in Hz for each electrode

The sensitivity of the spectrum can be changed by choosing FreqMapSen from the BmParam menu.

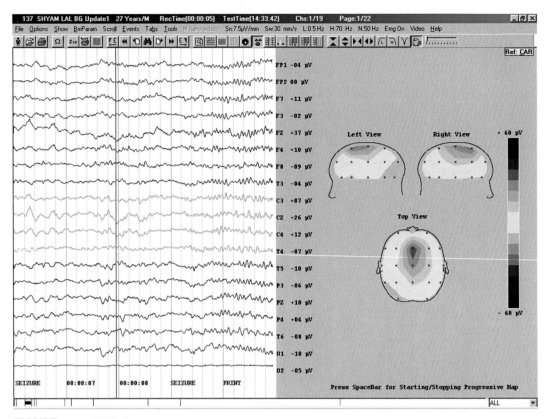

FIGURE 2.11   EEG trimap.

- **BmParam** contains several features, as described below.
  - **Reference**: To view the maps all electrodes must be considered with some reference. The following references are provided in the machine.
    - **CAR (common average reference)**: Average of standard 21 EEG electrodes.
    - **Linked ear**: Average of A1 and A2.
  - **FreqMapSen** helps in selecting the value of sensitivity for brain mapping. Options provided are 2, 4, 6, 10, 15, 20, 30, 40, 60, 100, 150, 200, 300, 400, 600, 1000, 1500, and 2000 μV^2/Hz.
- **Tools-Amplitude Progressive**: Fig. 2.14 shows maps for amplitude progression: 12 amplitude maps can be viewed consecutively with a time difference of 7.8125 ms. from the point when the EEG was clicked. These images have been considered for the research mentioned in chapter "Proposed EEG/Speech-Based Emotion Recognition System: A Case Study" of this book.
- **Tools-Frequency Progressive**: Fig. 2.15 shows frequency progression maps. The yellow bar of EEG trace represents 2 s of selected EEG signals. The right side shows frequency maps for bands definable by the user in the menu by clicking user frequency bands.
  - **User Frequency Bands**: Fig. 2.16 shows the user frequency bands. The user can define 12 bands to be used in progressive frequency maps.

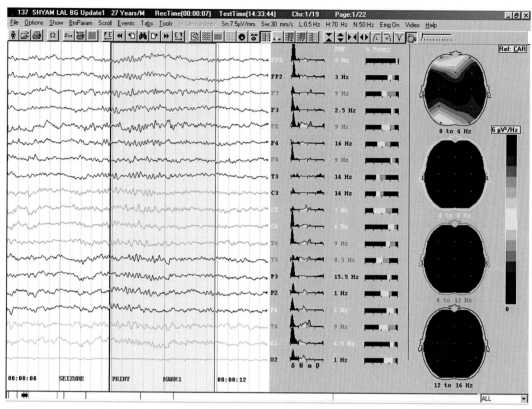

FIGURE 2.12   EEG frequency maps.

- **Tools-Frequency Tables**: The yellow bar of EEG trace shown in Fig. 2.17 represents 2 s of selected EEG signals for the frequency table. The right side shows a table for **absolute power**, **relative power**, **PPF**, and **MPF** for each electrode in each of the four frequency bands.

Some of the different tools available in Analysis software give information about signals, and some give information about images.[19]

2.5 ARTIFACTS

Artifacts are signals with no cerebral origin. They mainly have three origins: ocular, muscular, or mechanical. The artifact in the recorded EEG may be either patient/subject-related or technical. Patient/subject-related artifacts are unwanted physiological signals that may significantly disturb the EEG. Technical artifacts, such as AC power line noise, can be reduced by decreasing electrode impedance and using shorter electrode wires. The most common EEG artifact sources can be classified in the following ways.

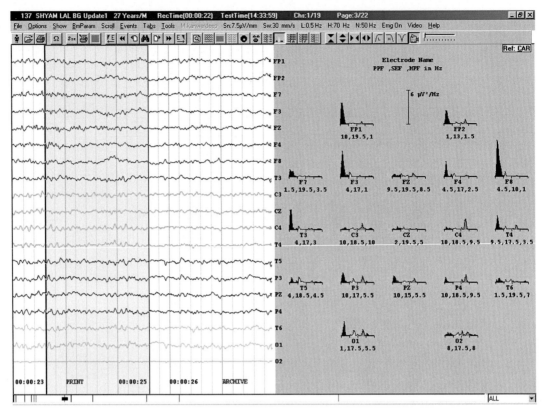

FIGURE 2.13   Frequency spectra maps.

- Subject related:
  - any minor body movements
  - ECG (pulse, pacemaker)
  - eye movements
  - sweating
- Technical related:
  - impedance fluctuation
  - cable movements
  - broken wire contacts
  - too much electrode paste/jelly or dried pieces
  - low battery

Some examples of artifacts during certain events are shown below.

2.5.1 Eye Blinks

Fig. 2.18 shows EEG signals related to eye blinks generating a slow signal (<4 Hz), corresponding to mechanical movement of the eyelid. The signal appears mainly in the frontal area (Fp1 and Fp2), and is symmetrical between the two hemispheres.

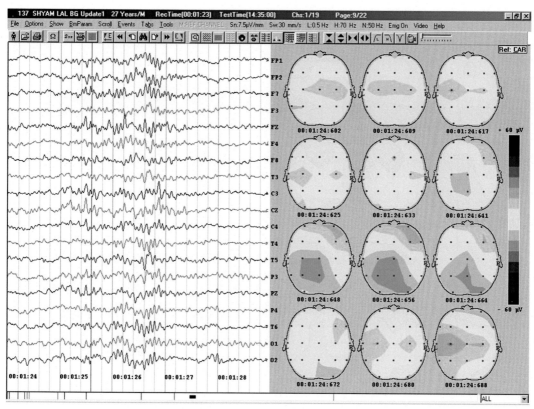

FIGURE 2.14   Amplitude progressive maps.

2.5.2 Eye Movement

Fig. 2.19 shows EEG signals related to eye movement that generates a slow signal (<4 Hz), corresponding to mechanical movement. The eyes make a dipole, which moves closer to or away from some electrodes and creates the signal. The signals appear mainly in the frontal and temporal areas, and are propagated more often than blinks. This signal is not symmetrical between the two hemispheres.

2.5.3 Muscular Artifacts

Fig. 2.20 shows EEG signals corresponding to muscular activity generating high frequency signals (>13 Hz), often much higher than cerebral signals. The main head muscle is the jaw, which can create an important signal in the temporal area (0–5 s). Frontal muscles can appear as well, since they are located just under the electrodes.

2.5.4 Electrode Artifacts

Fig. 2.21 presents EEG signals related to wire or electrode movements creating a low-frequency artifact (<2 Hz) on one electrode. The signal often has high amplitude. It is

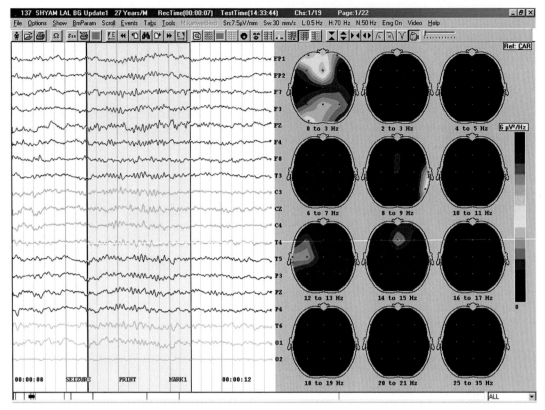

FIGURE 2.15   Frequency progressive maps.

also possible that a mechanical artifact will appear following a head movement, and in this case a signal appears on several electrodes.[20]

2.6 SPEECH ACQUISITION AND PROCESSING

Speech processing is the study of speech signals and processing methods. The signals are usually processed in a digital representation, so speech processing can be regarded as a special case of digital signal processing, applied to speech signals. Aspects of speech processing include the acquisition, manipulation, storage, transfer, and output of speech signals.

Speech processing has been defined as the study of speech signals and their processing methods, and also as the intersection of digital signal processing and natural language processing.

Speech processing technologies are used for digital speech coding, spoken language dialog systems, text-to-speech synthesis, and automatic speech recognition. Information (such as speaker, gender, or language identification, or speech recognition) can also be extracted from speech.

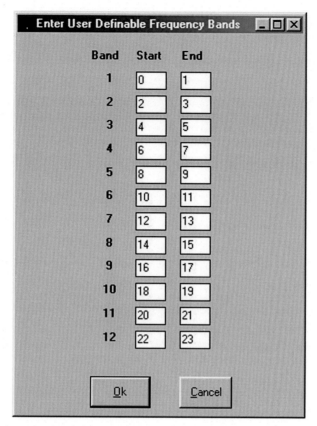

FIGURE 2.16   User frequency bands used in EEG.

Speech may be a more intuitive way of accessing information, controlling things, and communicating, but there may be viable alternatives: speech is not necessarily the "natural" way to interact with a computer. Speech is hands-free, eyes-free, fast, and intuitive.

Speech processing would be easier if there were simple linear relationships between articulations and acoustics, and between acoustics and perception. This would greatly facilitate automatic speech synthesis and recognition, respectively.[21]

2.6.1 Applications of Speech Recognition[22]

- Speech emotion recognition in intelligent household robots.
- Speaker verification.
- Speech identification on the basis of mood.
- Interactive voice response systems.
- Train reservation systems.
- Automation of operator services.
- Voice dialing.

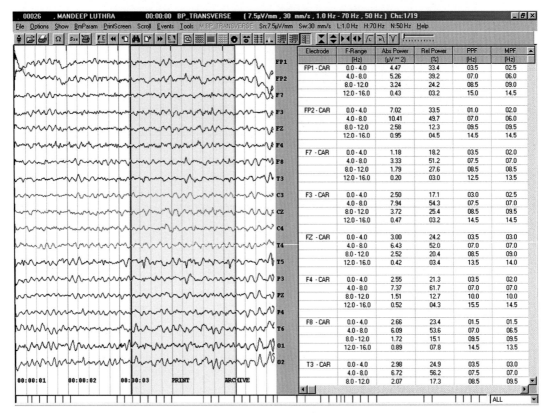

FIGURE 2.17   Frequency tables used in EEG.

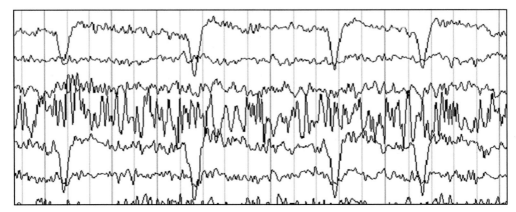

FIGURE 2.18   Artifacts for eye blinks seen in EEG signals.

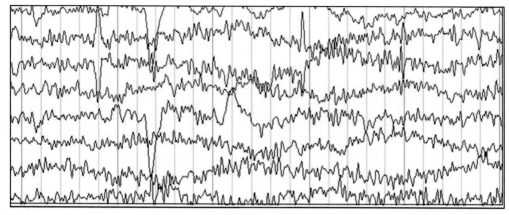

FIGURE 2.19   Artifacts for eye movements seen in EEG signals.

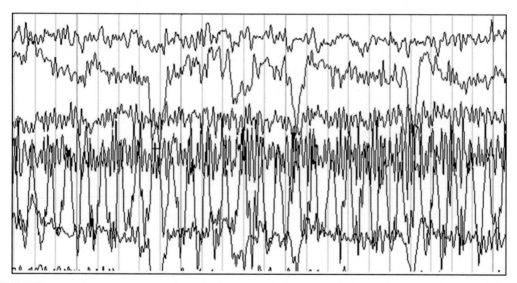

FIGURE 2.20   Artifacts for muscular movements seen in EEG signals.

- Voice navigation of a desktop.
- Call center automation.

2.6.2 Acquisition Setup

To achieve a high audio quality, generally speech acquisition is done in a normal room without noisy sound or echo effects. An appropriate sampling frequency needs to be selected: it is generally 16 KHz. The speakers are allowed to sit in front of the microphone at a distance of about 12—15 cm. The speech data was collected with the help of Computerized Speech

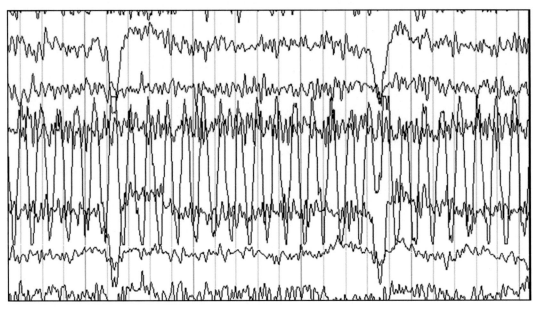

FIGURE 2.21   Artifacts for electrode movement.

Laboratory (CSL) using a single channel. CSL is the most advanced analysis system for speech and voice: it is an input/output recording device for a PC, with special features for reliable acoustic measurements.[23]

Speech signal acquisition is a very important step in speech processing. If the acquired signal is not properly recorded, the system performance will be reduced. Ideally, speech recordings should take place in soundproof studios or research labs. If those are not available, one should try to find a relatively quiet room with as little low-frequency noise as possible. Most typical sources of low-frequency noise include 60 Hz hum from electrical equipment, heating, and air-conditioning ducts, elevators, doors, water pipes, computer fans, and other mechanical systems in the building. If possible, these devices should be switched off during recording. For speech signal recording the government of India's Department of Linguistics has published the Linguistic Data Consortium for Indian Languages (LDC-IL) standard.[24] PRAAT, CSL, Audacity, Sphinx, and Julius are various tools which are being used by researchers for recording speech databases.[25,26]

2.7 COMPUTERIZED SPEECH LABORATORY

CSL is a highly advanced acoustic analysis system with robust hardware for data acquisition, complemented by the most versatile suite of software available for speech analysis, teaching, research, voice measurement, clinical feedback, acoustic phonetics, and forensic work.

The **KayPENTAX CSL model 4500**, an input/output audio device that meets the exacting specifications for reliable acoustic measurements in clinics and research labs, is described with its features.

2.7.1 Key Features of CSL

1. CSL is a four-channel input device which gives the ability to collect more signals simultaneously for reliable speech acquisition and analysis in the areas of research and clinical applications.
2. It provides AC and DC coupling, where AC couplings are used to remove low-frequency components for improved signal quality and DC inputs are used for low-frequency data signals such as electroglottography.
3. CSL offers signal-to-noise performance typically superior to generic sound cards.
4. It incorporates design features for accurate voice signal capture, such as use of low-latency audio stream input output drivers, high-gain preamplification, and antialias filtering.
5. CSL meets the exacting hardware standards defined by the National Center for Voice and Speech.
6. Higher sampling rates of 8000–200,000 Hz are allowed for analysis of higher-frequency signals for researchers in certain applications (eg, bioacoustics).

2.7.2 Facilities Available in CSL

2.7.2.1 Record and Speak Facilities

CSL has a facility to record and speak the input speech data (Fig. 2.22). The Record option is provided by the File menu, which also gives access to the various commands needed to load a signal from disk, save a signal from memory to disk, generate a waveform, select configuration files, print, and exit the program. The Speak menu gives access to commands related to speaking or playing the stored signal to speaker output.

- **New (Record)** helps to capture a signal through the selected input channel(s) and display the waveform in the active window. Characteristics of the recording, eg, number of channels, sampling rate, etc., are determined by the Capture options.
- **Speaking Data**: The program allows generation of audio output of waveform data. The program automatically associates a window containing analysis results data with its source waveforms. It also obtains audio output from analysis result data displayed over time. Users may speak all the data or a specified range of it, and can also specify two ranges within the data.
- **Open (Load)** loads sample data from a file and displays it as a graphic waveform in the empty active window.
- **Save** saves the waveform data in the active window in an audio file. The recorded data can be saved in various formats, such as CSL signal file format (**.NSP**) with a maximum of eight channels, wave and audio file format (**.WAV**) with a maximum of two channels, and (**.RAW**) audio file format without headers.

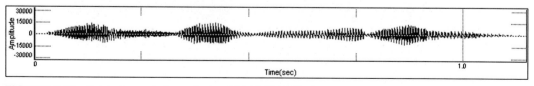

FIGURE 2.22 Original recorded speech signal "AAJ SUB NIRAV HAI."

- **Generating a Waveform**: The program allows creation of a waveform signal, with a number of parameters specified to control the waveform characteristics and display it in the active window. The signal may be generated in various forms, such as sine wave, square wave, triangular wave, sawtooth wave, or white noise. Start and end amplitude, frequency, sampling rate, phase angle, and duration of waveform can also set at a required specific value.
- **RESET (to the user configuration)** resets and accesses the parameter settings in the user configuration file.

2.7.2.2 Analytical Tools

The equipment includes a variety of analytical tools which are provided in the analysis menu (Fig. 2.23). All graphical analysis requires a window display. CSL includes functions to perform the following types of analysis on a waveform signal.

- **Linear Predictive Coding Analysis (LPC)** is used to generate a discrete LPC frequency response of a frame of sampled data starting at a specified location in the source window, and to display the resulting frequency response as a spectrum in the active window (Fig. 2.24).
- **LPC Waterfall Analysis (LPCW)** generates a series of LPC frequency responses, taking frames of waveform data in a specified range in the source window and displaying the resulting frequency responses in a waterfall array in the active window (Fig. 2.25).
- **Fast Fourier Transform Analysis (FFT)** generates a discrete power spectrum using the FFT algorithm of a frame of sampled data starting at a specified location of data in the source window, and displays the resulting power spectrum in the active window (Fig. 2.26).

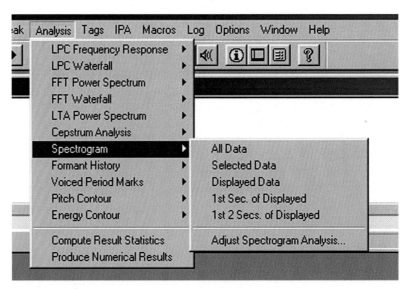

FIGURE 2.23   Analysis menu with selected spectrogram menu.

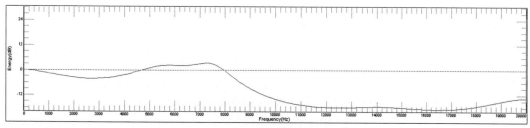

FIGURE 2.24   Linear predictive coding analysis of the original speech signal.

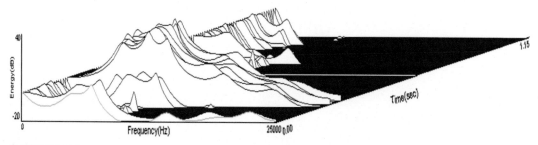

FIGURE 2.25   Linear predictive coding waterfall analysis of the original speech signal.

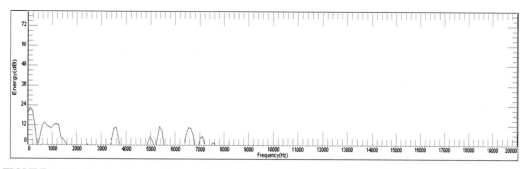

FIGURE 2.26   Fast Fourier transform analysis of the original speech signal.

- **FFT Waterfall Analysis (FFTW)** generates a series of FFT power spectra, displayed in a waterfall array (Fig. 2.27).
- **LTA Power Analysis (LTA)** generates a long-term average (LTA) power spectrum using the FFT algorithm (Fig. 2.28).
- **Cepstrum Analysis or Inverse Spectrum (CEPSTRUM)** helps to generate an inverse spectrum from a power spectrum that was previously generated with either the FFT or LTA commands (Fig. 2.29). The inverse spectrum is generated by taking an FFT of the log magnitude values of a power spectrum. The purpose of the inverse spectrum is to isolate the harmonic energy that is present in a spectrum of voiced speech, which can be used to determine the fundamental frequency of the voiced signal.

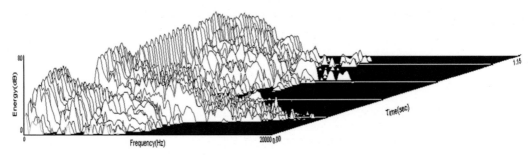

FIGURE 2.27   Fast Fourier transform waterfall analysis of the original speech signal.

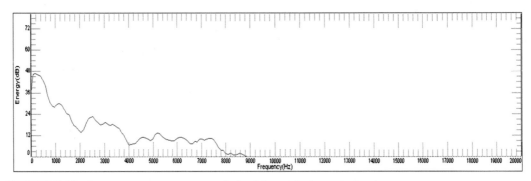

FIGURE 2.28   Long-term average power analysis of the original speech signal.

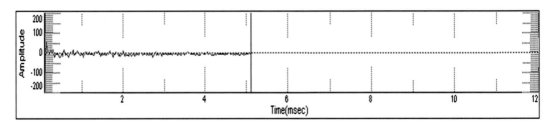

FIGURE 2.29   Cepstrum analysis or inverse spectrum (CEPSTRUM) of the original speech signal.

- **Spectrographic Analysis (SPG)** generates an FFT-based three-dimensional spectrogram (Fig. 2.30). A power spectrum is computed for a series of frames of sampled data in a specified range. Each computed spectrum is displayed as a single vertical column, with frequency on the vertical axis and time represented on the horizontal axis. The energy is expressed in darkness or color gradients.
- **Formant History (FMT)** generates an LPC-based formant display over time (Fig. 2.31).
- **Impulse Marks (Voiced Period Marks or IMPULSE)** is used to compute and mark the locations separating voice periods in speech waveform data. The process separates the voiced signal into its periodic components, the inverse of each period being the fundamental frequency, or pitch separation of the signal as it changes over time (Fig. 2.32).

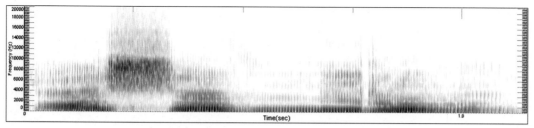

FIGURE 2.30   Spectrographic analysis of the original speech signal.

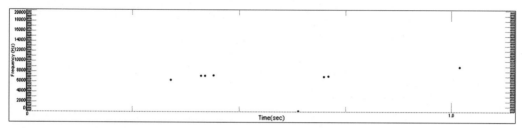

FIGURE 2.31   Formant history of the original speech signal.

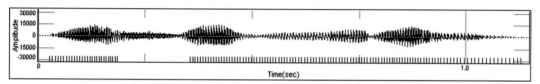

FIGURE 2.32   Impulse marks (Voiced Period Marks or IMPULSE) of the original speech signal.

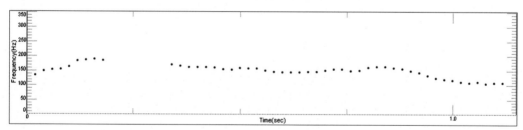

FIGURE 2.33   Pitch contour (PITCH) of the original speech signal.

- **Pitch Contour (PITCH)** computes the fundamental frequency (pitch) of voice speech data (Fig. 2.33).
- **Energy Contour (ENERGY)** is used to perform an energy calculation (Fig. 2.34). The energy operation calculates the sum of the absolute amplitude values in a frame of data divided by the number of points in the frame. The energy is first computed and then converted to decibels of sound pressure (dB SPL).

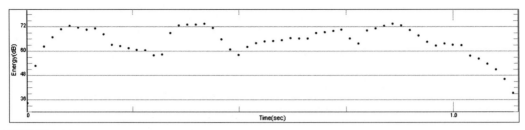

FIGURE 2.34   Energy contour (ENERGY) of the original speech signal.

- **Compute Result Statistics**: The program provides facilities to display, print and save a series of statistical analyses that are derived from the most recently commuted analysis results in the active window.
- **Produce Numerical Results** displays numerical results of the last analysis performed.

2.7.2.3 Other Special Features

CSL also has many special features in various available menus, such as edit, log, view, IPA, macros, option, etc. Some of these are described below.

- **Data types**. Three types of data exist in the graphics work environment of a program window: waveform data, analysis data, and transient data.
  - **Waveform data** provides the basis for all other types of program data. All audio data that is captured by the program using an A/D conversion is stored in binary format as numerical values. These numerical values may be displayed in graphic format and played back as audio data using digital-to-analog conversion. Waveform data displayed in graphic format has time represented along the horizontal axis and amplitude displayed along the vertical axis.
  - **Analysis data** provides analysis operations which may be performed once waveform data has been displayed in the source window. The analysis data can be saved to a file for later processing or plotting, except for the spectrogram and waterfall arrays.
  - **Transient data** is the spectrogram, the FFT waterfall array, and the LPC waterfall array. Transient data is nothing but the output of an analysis calculation, which is not supported by numerical results or statistics. This data cannot be saved to file.
- **Filter Source Data**: A finite impulse response (FIR) digital filter can be applied to a specified range of waveform data in the source window and the resulting filtered waveform copied to the active window. Users can build an FIR digital filter file using the parameters selected. The frequency response will be displayed in the response window. Before applying it to the sampled data, the filter coefficients of a recently build filter must be saved to disk or an existing digital filter loaded from disk. The most recently saved or loaded filter will be applied to the waveform data. The filter source data option is specified in the edit menu.
- **Adjust Signal Offset**: The program provides a facility to remove any DC offset or float that may be generated by a multimedia card. The DC offset value may be calculated automatically from the waveform data and subtracted from the amplitude values in the data, or a manually specified offset value may be applied.

- **Down-sample Display Source**: The program provides the facility for down-sampling a range of sampled data. It is typically used to reduce the sampling rate of a waveform after it has been filtered. The combination and filtering may be used to remove possible alias effects from digitally encoded waveform data.
- **Log menu**: The program offers the ability to record information taken from the cursor location and save it in an ASCII text file, called a log book. The log menu provides various functions, such as opening an existing or a new log file, setting up a new results log, closing the log book, etc.
- **Capture**: A capture signal option feature is provided in the option menu which specifies the various options for capturing the input data, such as active channel, sampling rate, capture length, etc., and also provides input device options for specific data acquisition hardware options.
- **Option menu** also provides access to many adjustments within the program for waveform, speak, editing, and especially for analysis functions.[27]

2.8 CONCLUSION

In this chapter we discuss the acquisitions of brain and speech signals and their processing through EEG and sound recording systems, respectively. To capture the signals of brain EEG, the imaging technique is useful. Due to technological advances, EEG equipment has moved from wired to wireless. This chapter discusses the merits and demerits of both types of systems. Brain signals are acquired with the help of electrodes. The American standard for placing these electrodes is implemented in acquisition. As an example of EEG equipment the RMS EEG 32-channel machine is explored, with its acquisition and analysis facilities. For speech signals, CSL is discussed. The chapter concludes with illustration of CSL and its utilities.

References

1. Niedermeyer E, Lopes da Silva FH. *Electroencephalography: Basic Principles, Clinical Applications and Related Fields.* 3rd ed. Philadelphia: Lippincott, Williams & Wilkins; 1993.
2. Atwood HL, MacKay WA. *Essentials of Neurophysiology.* 1989. Canada.
3. Tyner FS, Knott JR. *Fundamentals of EEG Technology.* In: *Basic Concepts and Methods.* Vol. 1. New York: Raven Press; 1989.
4. Nunez PL. *Neocortical Dynamics and Human EEG Rhythms.* New York: Oxford University Press; 1995.
5. *Electroencephalogram.* http://www.eelab.usyd.edu.au/ELEC3801/notes/Electroencephalogram.htm.
6. Cohen D. Magnetoencephalography. In: Adelman G, ed. *Encyclopedia of Neuroscience.* Cambridge, USA: Birkhauser; 1987:601–604.
7. Bronzino JD. Principles of electroencephalography. In: Bronzino JD, ed. *The Biomedical Engineering Handbook.* Florida: CRC Press; 1995:201–212.
8. Fralich T. *Emotions, Mindfulness and the Pathways of the Brain.* http://www.belmont.edu/studentaffairs/pdfs_and_images/emotions.pdf.
9. Teplan M. *Fundamentals of EEG Measurement.* In: *Measurement Science Review.* Vol. 2. 2002 (Section 2).
10. ZIfkin BG. Clinical neurophysiology with special reference to the electroencephalogram. *Giullano Avanzini Epilepsis.* 2009;50(suppl):30–38.
11. *Grass technologies EEG Products.* http://www.grasstechnologies.com/products/clinsystems/cmxleeg-plus1.html.
12. *StatNet EEG Equipment.* http://www.hydrodot.net/Products/statnet.html.

13. Lee S, Shin Y, Woo S, Kim K, Lee HN. *Review of Wireless Brain-Computer Interface Systems, Brain-Computer Interface Systems — Recent Progress and Future Prospects.* InTech; 2013. http://dx.doi.org/10.5772/56436. ISBN 978-953-51-1134-4.
14. Effects of Electrode Placement. http://www.focused-technology.com/electrod.htm.
15. Collura T. *A Guide to Electrode Selection, Location and Application for EEG Biofeedback.* 1998. Ohio.
16. Kondraske GV. Neurophysiologic measurements. In: Bronzino JD, ed. *Biomedical Engineering and Instrumentation.* Boston: PWS Publishing; 1986:138—179.
17. *RMS EEG Machine.* http://www.rmsindia.com/.
18. *Help Manual of EEG Acquire Software.* http://www.rmsindia.com/.
19. *Help Manual of EEG Analysis Software.* http://www.rmsindia.com/.
20. *Artifacts.* http://www.samuelboudet.com/en/EEG/artefacts.php.
21. Deng L, O'Shaughnessy D. *Speech Processing a Dynamic and Optimization-Oriented Approach.* June 2003. New York.
22. *Applications of Speech Recognition.* https://en.wikipedia.org/wiki/Speech_recognition.
23. Gaikwad S, Gawali B, Yannawar P. Performance analysis of MFCC & DTW for isolated arabic digit. *Int J Adv Res Comput Sci.* 2011;2(1).
24. *Linguistics Data Consortium for Indian languages.* http://www.ldcil.org/.
25. *The Disordered Voice Database.* Available: http://www.kayelemetrics.com/Product%20Info/CSL%20Family/4500/4500.htm.
26. Mathur R, Babita, Kansal A. Domain specific speaker independent continuous speech recognizer using Julius. In: *Proceedings of ASCNT.* Noida, India: CDAC; 2010:55—60.
27. *Manual for Computerized Speech Laboratory (CSL) Machine.* http://kayelemetrics.com/index.php?option=com_product&Itemid=3&controller=product&task=learn_more&cid[]=11.

Technical Aspects of Brain Rhythms and Speech Parameters

3.1 INTRODUCTION TO BRAIN-WAVE FREQUENCIES

The electrical activity in the brain depends upon the type of activity being done by a person. For example, the brain waves of a person who is reading are very different to those of a person who is relaxing.[1,2] These brain waves/rhythms are classified in five categories, and provide information about a person's health and state of mind.[3] The categories are described in the following subsections.

3.1.1 Gamma Waves

A gamma wave is considered to be the fastest brain activity. It is responsible for cognitive functioning, learning, memory, and information processing. Prominence of this wave leads

Introduction to EEG- and Speech-Based Emotion Recognition
http://dx.doi.org/10.1016/B978-0-12-804490-2.00003-8

to anxiety, high arousal, and stress; while its suppression can lead to Attention Deficit Hyperactivity Disorder (ADHD), depression, and learning disabilities. In optimal conditions gamma waves help with attention, focus, binding of senses (smell, sight, and hearing), consciousness, mental processing, and perception.[4]

3.1.2 Beta Waves

Beta waves are high-frequency, low-amplitude brain waves that are commonly observed in an awaken state. They are involved in conscious thought and logical thinking, and tend to have a stimulating effect. Having the right amount of beta waves allows us to focus. Prominence of this wave causes anxiety, high arousal, an inability to relax, and stress, whereas its suppression can lead to ADHD, daydreaming, depression, and poor cognition. In optimal conditions beta waves help with conscious focus, memory, and problem solving. These waves can be divided into three specific classifications.[5]

- **Low beta waves (12–15 Hz)**: known as "beta one" waves and associated mostly with quiet, focused, introverted concentration.
- **Mid-range beta waves (15–20 Hz)**: known as "beta two" waves and associated with increases in energy, anxiety, and performance.
- **High beta waves (18–40 Hz)**: known as "beta three" waves and associated with significant stress, anxiety, paranoia, high energy, and high arousal.

3.1.3 Alpha Waves

Alpha waves have a frequency range between beta and theta. They help us calm down when necessary and promote feelings of deep relaxation. Alpha waves are found prominently in daydreaming, inability to focus, and being very relaxed. If they are suppressed it can cause anxiety, high stress, and insomnia. When they are optimal it leads to a relaxed state.[6]

3.1.4 Theta Waves

This particular frequency range is involved in daydreaming and sleep. ADHD, depression, hyperactivity, impulsivity, and inattentiveness are observed when theta waves are prominent; if they are suppressed, anxiety, poor emotional awareness, and stress can be seen. In an optimal state, theta helps in creativity, emotional connection, intuition, and relaxation. Theta waves have benefits of helping to improve our intuition and creativity, and making us feel more natural. Theta is also involved in restorative sleep.[7]

3.1.5 Delta Waves

Delta waves are the slowest recorded brain waves in human beings. They are found most often in infants and young children, and are associated with the deepest levels of relaxation and restorative, healing sleep. Delta is prominently seen in brain injuries, learning problems, inability to think, and severe ADHD. If this wave is suppressed, it leads to an inability to rejuvenate the body and revitalize the brain, and poor sleep. Adequate production of delta waves helps us feel completely rejuvenated and promotes the immune system, natural healing, and restorative/deep sleep.[8]

Fig. 3.1 shows the data band of an EEG of 2 s duration with its absolute power values for δ, θ, α, and β signals.

3.2 SPEECH PROSODIC FEATURES

Prosodic information plays an important role in the human speech recognition process. Prosody can be identified with different levels of data from phonetic, paralinguistic and nonphonetic.[9]

The investigation of emotional expression in the voice depends on feelings depicted in words and their way of pronunciation. These variations in acoustic changes are because of different levels of normal to physiological excitement for distinctive feelings. Along these lines estimations of the acoustic properties of angry, happy and fearful emotions have raised excitement levels.[10]

3.2.1 Acoustic Features for Emotions

Emotional expression and understanding are normal instincts of human beings, but automatic emotion recognition from speech without referring any language or linguistic information remains an unclosed problem. The most widespread acoustic features are mainly based on models of the human auditory system.[11] The acoustic features related to emotion recognition task are classified as:

3.2.1.1 *Prosody-Related Signal Measures*

Emotional states are correlated with particular physiological states, which in turn have mechanical and predictable effects on speech, especially on pitch (fundamental frequency F_0), timing, and voice quality.[12] The most affected prosodic features for emotion are:[13,14]

- energy
- pitch
- formant
- intensity
- loudness
- duration
- sampling rate.

3.2.1.1.1 ENERGY

The energy is the basic and most important feature in a speech signal. It plays an important role in the performance of acoustic model-based emotion recognition. The energy of speech is

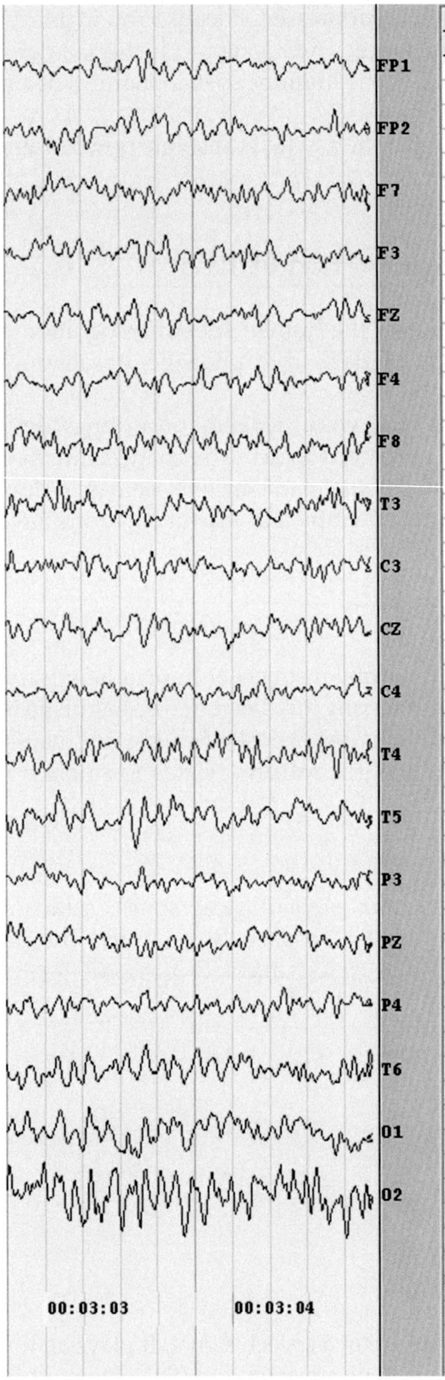

Electrode	F-Range (Hz)	Abs Power (µV ** 2)
FP1 - CAR	δ	4.20
	θ	2.29
	α	6.70
	β	3.37
FP2 - CAR	δ	5.72
	θ	4.17
	α	6.77
	β	2.24
F7 - CAR	δ	6.95
	θ	1.94
	α	2.86
	β	0.64
F3 - CAR	δ	4.08
	θ	4.54
	α	11.63
	β	1.96
FZ - CAR	δ	2.78
	θ	8.53
	α	7.55
	β	2.34
F4 - CAR	δ	4.82
	θ	4.19
	α	5.10
	β	2.68
F8 - CAR	δ	4.90
	θ	4.33
	α	7.02
	β	2.06
T3 - CAR	δ	33.79
	θ	1.72
	α	2.41
	β	4.26
C3 - CAR	δ	2.34
	θ	2.69
	α	5.28
	β	2.46
CZ - CAR	δ	5.35
	θ	11.80
	α	5.50
	β	1.88
C4 - CAR	δ	2.99
	θ	3.20
	α	2.72
	β	1.37

FIGURE 3.1   EEG 2 s data band with absolute power values for δ, θ, α, and β signals.

a basic and independent parameter. The energy of each frame is calculated by Eq. [3.1] as follows.

$$E_t = \int_t^{t+r} |X[t]|^2 dt \qquad\qquad [3.1]$$

At time t where E_i is the energy of the ith frame with duration t and $|X[t]|$ is the amplitude of the signal at time t. $|\ |$ means modules of amplitude.

The energy of all the frames is ordered and the top ones are selected to obtain the pitch features. The voiced frame is determined by calculating the energy contained within certain bandwidths. A simple energy calculation is able to yield speech frames which contain a relatively strong pitch feature. The amplitude of unvoiced segments is noticeably lower than that of the voiced segments. The short-time energy of speech signals reflects the amplitude variation.[15] The graphical representation of energy feature in speech signal is shown in Fig. 3.2. We can obtain the statistics of energy with the mean value, maximum value, variance, variation range, and contour of energy.

Combination of the loudness recognition with the acoustic estimation is as complex as the tone's coupling pitch discernment and the process able F_0. The sensation of loudness is dependent on both the frequency of sound and duration. The pitch perception depends on loudness. Thus, precise, complex dependence is not specifically considered for accompanying calculation, energy and F_0 figuring are put away in a vector for an implicit standardization.[16]

Basic calculation procedures used for computation of energy as the acoustic correlated of perceptual loudness are based on relations between physical acoustic pressure magnitudes p_s,

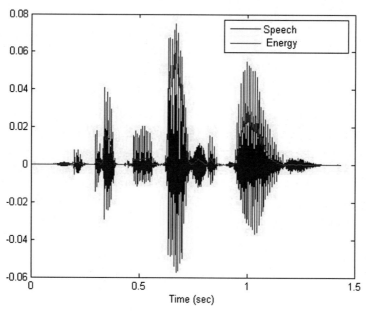

FIGURE 3.2   Representation of energy feature in speech signal.

measured in Pascal ($1\text{Pa} = 1\,\text{N/m}^2$), and the acoustic intensity I_s, which unit is W/m^2. It can be stated that I_s is proportional to p_s. With the help of the acoustic intensity reference value, $I_0 = 1\,_p\text{W/m}^2$, and the acoustic pressure reference value, $p_0 = 20\,\mu\text{Pa}$, which illustrates the human auditory threshold at mid-range frequencies, the absolute acoustic pressure in decibels (dB) is given by

$$L = 10 \cdot \log \frac{I_s}{I_0} \, \text{dB} = 20 \cdot \log \frac{p_s}{p_0} \, \text{dB} \qquad [3.2]$$

The acoustic magnitude loudness quantifies the sound intensity rate between two perceived tones, hence a sound of 1 kHz with a loudness of 40 phones (acoustic pressure level of 40 dB) is applied as reference. Automatic computation of energy contour can be achieved through different methods. A general method is employed using the Eq. [3.3].

$$E_m = \sum_{n=-\infty}^{n=\infty} T(s_n) w_{m-n} \qquad [3.3]$$

T represents a convenient transformation of signal values s_n and w_n that corresponds to an adequate window function to obtain precise segments of the signal. Values that fall out of the window are set to 0, in order to facilitate finite procedures. There are many possibilities for the choice of the transformation and the windowing function. In the loudness calculation process, a Hamming window has been used w_n^H with the form

$$w_n^H = 0.54 - 0.46 \cos\left(\frac{2\pi n}{N-1}\right) \qquad [3.4]$$

For the loudness calculation, the reference value I_0 is needed, which can no longer be extracted from digitized signals. For a 16-bit quantization and a maximum acoustic pressure level of 60 dB, represents a standard value during normal conversation, I_0 is computed by Eq. [3.5] as follows:

$$Lh_i = 10 \cdot \log \frac{(2^{15})^2}{I_0} = 60 \, \text{dB} \rightarrow \overline{I}_0 = \frac{(2^{15})^2}{10^6} \approx 1073.74 \qquad [3.5]$$

Using Hamming windows w_n^H of 40 ms of duration, thus with 40 ms/16,000/s = 640 samples ($N = 640$), the intensity value I_s of the frame i can be estimated through the Eq. [3.6].

$$\widetilde{I}_i = \frac{\sum_{n=0}^{639} s_{i+n}^2 \cdot w_n^H}{\sum_{n=0}^{639} w_n^H} \qquad [3.6]$$

The effective loudness value Lh_i of the frame i can therefore be estimated through its relation to the intensity as in Eq. [3.7].

$$Lh_i = \sqrt[3]{\frac{\widetilde{I}_i}{\overline{I}_0}} \qquad [3.7]$$

The energy related features are explained in Table 3.1.

TABLE 3.1   Detail Energy Related Feature for Emotion Recognition

Sr. No	Feature	Name	Description
1	ENER_MAX	Short-term energy maximum	Refers to maximum value of the energy curve in the whole utterance
2	ENER_MAX_POS	Position of short-term-energy maximum	Refers to relative time position of the maximum energy value into the utterance
3	ENER_MIN	Short-term-energy minimum	Refers to minimum value of the energy curve into the whole utterance
4	ENER_MIN_POS	Position of short-term-energy minimum	Refers to relative time position of the minimum energy value into the utterance
5	ENER_REG_COEF	Regression coefficient for short-term-energy	Refers to slope coefficient of the regression line for the energy curve values in the utterance
6	ENER SQR_ERR	Mean square error for regression coefficient for short-term-energy	Refers to mean square error value between the regression line and the real energy curve
7	ENER_MEAN	Mean of short-term-energy	Refers to mean energy value calculated over the whole utterance
8	ENER_VAR	Variance of short-term-energy	Refers to Variance of the energy values over the whole utterance

3.2.1.1.2 PITCH

Pitch which is the main acoustic correlation of tone and intonation, it gives highest peak of the wave by which we can recognize the state of emotions. Fundamental frequency (F_0) estimation, also referred as pitch detection, has been a popular research topic for many years, and is still being investigated today. The basic period is called the pitch period. The average pitch frequency time pattern, gain, and fluctuation change from one individual speaker to another. The pitch detector's algorithm[17] can be given by Eqs. [3.8] and [3.9]. Fig. 3.3 describes a vocal phoneme, in which the pitch marks are denoted in red.

$$\langle x, y \rangle = \int_{t_0}^{t_0+r} x(t) \cdot y(t) dt; \quad y(t) = x(t-r) \tag{3.8}$$

Where $x(t)$ and $y(t)$ are vocal phoneme parameters.

$$p_r = \frac{\langle x, y \rangle}{||x|| \cdot ||y||}; \quad ||x|| = (\langle x, x \rangle)^2 \tag{3.9}$$

where $x(t)$ is signal at time t pitch $T_0 = \arg(\max(Pr))$.

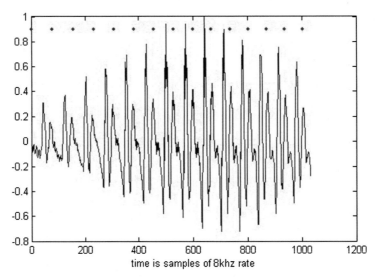

FIGURE 3.3   Graphical representation of pitch cycle in speech signal.

Current speech recognition engines often discard the pitch information as irrelevant to the recognition task. Much semantic information is passed on through pitch that is above the phonetic and lexical levels. In tonal languages, the relative pitch motion of an utterance contributes to the lexical information in a word.[18] Pitch is loosely related to the log of the frequency.[19,20] Pitch perception also changes with intensity, duration and other physical features of the waveform. The visual representation of pitch counter in speech signal is shown in Fig. 3.4.

The pitch based feature for emotion recognition is explained in Table 3.2.

3.2.1.1.3 FORMANT

Formant was stated by Gunnar Fant's in 1960. A formant is also referred as acoustic resonance of the human vocal tract. The spectral peaks of the spectrum are referred as formant. This definition is generally utilized in acoustic analysis and trade. The peaks that are determined within the spectrum envelope are referred to as formant.[21] In the process of formant,[22] it defines resonance frequencies of the vocal tract in terms of a gain operate $T(f)$ of the vocal tract: The frequency location of a maximum in $|T(f)|$. The resonance and formant are so conceptually distinct. The acoustics of the vocal tract are usually sculptured employing a mathematical model of a filter.[23] The frequencies of the poles of this filter model fall near those of the formant. The graphical representation of formant feature is shown in Fig. 3.5.

Formants are frequency peaks in the spectrum which have a high degree of energy. They are especially prominent in vowels. Each formant corresponds to a resonance in the vocal tract (roughly speaking, the spectrum has a formant every 1000 Hz). Formants can be considered as filters. Due to the joint resonance effect of the vocal cavities, filtering of sound takes

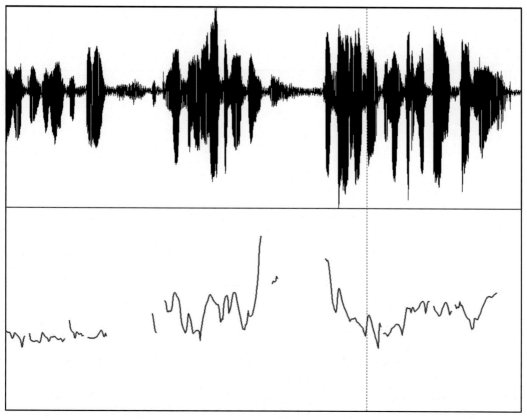

FIGURE 3.4   Representation of pitch values in speech signals.

place in the source sound, strengthening some frequency components (some harmonics) and attenuating others. The envelop of formant is described in Fig. 3.6.

3.2.1.1.4 INTENSITY

It is a measure of the radiated power (covered above) per unit area. Intensity decreases as the distance from the sound source increases, since the area through which the sound is being sent grows ever larger. Three distinct ways to control the loudness, or intensity are:

- changes made above the larynx (adjustments in the vocal tract)
- changes made in the larynx (activity in the laryngeal muscles)
- changes made below the larynx (breath control, changing lung pressure)

The representation of intensity value in speech signal is shown in Fig. 3.7.

TABLE 3.2   Pitch Features for Emotion Recognition[14]

Sr. No	Feature	Name
1	Feature 1	Pitch maximum gradient
2	Feature 2	Pitch relative position of maximum
3	Feature 3	Pitch standard deviation
4	Feature 4	Pitch mean value gradient
5	Feature 5	Pitch mean value
6	Feature 6	Pitch relative maximum
7	Feature 7	Pitch range
8	Feature 8	Pitch relative position of minimum
9	Feature 9	Pitch relative absolute area
10	Feature 10	Pitch relative minimum
11	Feature 11	Pitch mean distance between reversal points
12	Feature 12	Pitch standard dev. of dist. between reversal points

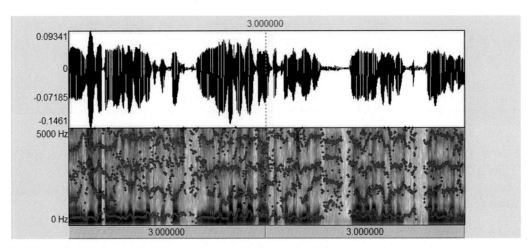

FIGURE 3.5   Graphical representation of formant feature in speech signal.

3.2.1.1.5 LOUDNESS

A perceptual quantity is assessed by an auditory system, including the brain. Perceived "loudness" varies according to pitch, because the human ear is not uniformly sensitive to all frequencies. For instance, the ear is most sensitive to pitches in the 1000—3000 Hz range. Lower or higher pitches, even if sung/produced at the same volume, will sound softer by comparison.

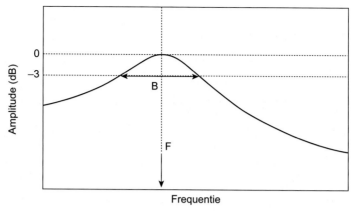

FIGURE 3.6   Envelop of formant in emotion recognition.

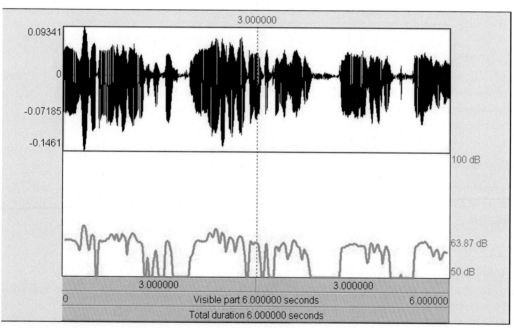

FIGURE 3.7   Representation of intensity values in speech signal.

3.2.1.1.6 DURATION

The duration feature plays an important role in the emotion recognition. The detail of duration based feature is explained in Table 3.3.

3.2.1.1.7 SAMPLING RATE

The sampling rate of speech recording also plays an important role. The variation of sampling rate is 8000, 16,000, 24,000, and 44,500 Hz.

TABLE 3.3   Duration Based Feature for Emotion Recognition[14]

Sr. No	Feature	Name
1	Feature 1	Duration mean value of voiced sounds
2	Feature 2	Duration of silences media
3	Feature 3	Duration of voiced sounds standard deviation

3.2.1.2 *Spectral Characteristics Measures*

Spectral characteristics are related to the harmonic/resonant structures resulting from the airflow modulated by dynamic vocal tract configurations. The classification of spectral characteristics measures are given below.

- Mel-frequency cepstral coefficients (MFCCs)
- Mel-filter bank energy slope feature (MFBs)

3.2.1.2.1 MEL-FREQUENCY CEPSTRAL COEFFICIENTS

MFCC is the robust and dynamic technique for speech feature extraction. There are 13 universally defined features computed using MFCC. These features are known as MFCC features. Researchers used the variation of MFCC feature for their experimentation.

13 MFCC feature (original)
26 MFCC feature (orignal + first derivative)
39 MFCC feature (original along with first and second derivative)

Implementation of MFCC technique resulted in 13 MFCC features where energy is the first feature followed by variation of energy.[24] The detail extracted MFCC features is explained the Table 3.4.

3.2.1.2.2 MEL FILTER BANK ENERGY BASED SLOPE FEATURES

It is a typical short-term spectral analysis technique, where speech data is split into overlapping time frames and spectrum of each frame is analyzed with DFT. Sub-band log-energies are computed with filters placed on Mel scale. It is premised that such analyses would emphasize formants in the spectrum, thus extracting speaker characteristics in that frame. Especially, higher level formants, that are known to be important in speech recognition, would gain importance during modeling. To overcome the effects of the channel, the mean of filterbank energies is subtracted out in the spectral domain. Since, the derivative of the spectral energies (in terms of least square fit) is computed; the zero crossing information gives formant information. The slope of the derivative is indicative of the bandwidth formant. Further, if two speakers have identical formant structure, the slope could perhaps be emphasizing the glottal pulse shape.[25] The detail of energy based slope feature is shown in Table 3.5.

TABLE 3.4 Detail of MFCC Feature for Emotion Recognition

Sr. No	Features	Name of feature
1	Feature 1	Energy
2	Feature 2	Energy of first level decomposed band
3	Feature 3	Energy intensity
4	Feature 4	Energy entropy
5	Feature 5	Energy for sub band
6	Feature 6	Jitter
7	Feature 7	Timbre
8	Feature 8	Duration
9	Feature 9	Average duration of every successive energy
10	Feature 10	Energy duration (original and decomposed band)
11	Feature 11	Gain of sampling frequency
12	Feature 12	Energy first band
13	Feature 13	Energy second band

TABLE 3.5 Energy Based Slope Feature for Emotion Recognition

Sr. No	Feature	Name of feature
1	Feature 1	Energy
2	Feature 2	Log of energy
3	Feature 3	Formant bandwidth
4	Feature 4	Energy slope

3.2.1.3 Voice Quality-related Measures

The classification of emotions using quality voice features is an emerging field of investigation, which is being used and referred in many lately studies concerned to emotion recognition.[26] The details of voice quality related measure are given below.

- Jitter
- Shimmer
- Harmonic-to-noise ratio

3.2.1.3.1 JITTER

Jitter is a measure of period-to-period fluctuations in fundamental frequency. It is calculated between consecutive voiced periods via the formula. Periodic jitter is defined as the relative mean absolute third-order difference of the point process. This feature is exceptionally calculated using Praat and then included in the feature vector.[27] The algorithm is computed through the formula explained in Eq. [3.10].

$$\text{jitter} = \frac{\sum_{i=2}^{N-1} |2 \cdot T_i - T_{i-1} - T_{i+1}|}{\sum_{i=2}^{N-1} T_i} \tag{3.10}$$

where, T_i = interval ith, N = number of intervals.

The variation of jitter features are shown in Table 3.6.

3.2.1.3.2 SHIMMER

Shimmer is defined as perturbations of the glottal source signal that occurs during vowel formation and affects glottal energy.[29] The features and measurement of shimmer feature is described as[28]

- Shimmer (dB) is expressed as the variability of the peak-to-peak amplitude in decibels, ie, the average absolute base-10 logarithm of the difference between the amplitudes of consecutive periods, multiplied by 20.
- Shimmer (relative) is defined as the average absolute difference between the amplitudes of consecutive periods, divided by the average amplitude, expressed as a percentage.
- Shimmer (apq3) is the three-point Amplitude Perturbation Quotient, the average absolute difference between the amplitude of a period and the average of the amplitudes of its neighbors, divided by the average amplitude.
- Shimmer (apq5) is defined as the five-point Amplitude Perturbation Quotient, the average absolute difference between the amplitude of a period and the average of the amplitudes of it and its four closest neighbors, divided by the average amplitude.

TABLE 3.6   Variation of Jitter Feature for Emotion Recognition[28]

Sr. No	Feature	Name of feature	Explanation
1	Feature 1	Jitter (absolute)	It is the cycle-to-cycle variation of fundamental frequency.
2	Feature 2	Jitter (relative)	It is the average absolute difference between consecutive periods, divided by the average period.
3	Feature 3	Jitter (rap)	It is defined as the relative average perturbation, the average absolute difference between a period and the average of it and its two neighbors, divided by the average period.
4	Feature 4	Jitter (ppq5)	It is the five-point period perturbation Quotient.

- Shimmer (apq11) is expressed as the 11-point Amplitude Perturbation Quotient, the average absolute difference between the amplitude of a period and the average of the amplitudes of it and its 10 closest neighbors, divided by the average amplitude.

3.2.1.3.3 HARMONIC TO NOISE RATIO

Harmonic to noise ratio is clearly related to the voice quality, this voice quality attribute has been said to provide valuable information about the speaker emotional state.[30] Harmonic to noise ratio estimation can be considered as an acoustic correlate for breathiness and roughness. Therefore, voice quality cues, which help us to infer assumptions about the speaker's emotional state, can be extracted from this attribute.

A common way of describing emotions is by assigning labels to them like emotion denoting words. There are a number of researchers that have compiled lists of emotional words. Of course some of these terms are more central to a certain emotion than others. Also, different emotion theories have different methods for selecting such basic emotion words. For recognition of emotions, the estimated parameters values obtained for five affects: calm, anger, sadness, happiness, comfort. Researcher got these parameters first by taking a gander at studies depicting the acoustic relates of every emotion, then concluded some starting quality for the parameters and changed them by hand, by experimentation until it gave a wonderful result. These outcomes give us a model of intonation contours for the different emotions:[12]

- **Happiness**: The mean pitch of the utterance is high, has a high variance, the rhythm is rather fast, few syllables are accented, the last word is accented, and the contours of all syllables are rising.
- **Anger**: The mean pitch is high, has a high variance, the rhythm is fast, with little variety of phoneme durations, a lot of syllables are accented, the last word is not accented, the pitch contours of all syllables are falling.
- **Sadness**: The mean pitch is low, has a low variance, the rhythm is slow, with high variance of phoneme durations, very few syllables are accented, the last word is not accented, the contours of all syllables are falling.
- **Comfort**: The mean pitch is high, but less than happy, the rhythm is slow, with a high variance of phoneme durations, very few syllables are accented, the last syllable is accented, and the contours of syllables are rising.

3.3 SIGNAL PROCESSING ALGORITHMS

BCI systems that use non-movement assumes that different mental tasks (eg, solving a multiplication problem, imagining a 3D object, or mental counting, emotion related responses) leads to distinct, task-specific distribution of EEG frequency patterns over the scalp patterns and aim to detect the patterns associated with these mental tasks from the EEG. To detect and analyze these patterns various signal processing algorithms are employed. The algorithms are divided into three categories they are:[31]

- Preprocessing
- Feature extraction/dimensionality reduction
- Feature classification

3.3.1 Preprocessing Algorithms

The processing performed on raw data and preparing, it for further processing refers to preprocessing. Different tools and methods implemented for preprocessing, includes[32]:

- **Sampling**: which selects a representative subset from a large population of data?
- **Transformation**: which manipulates raw data to produce a single input
- **De-noising**: which removes noise from data
- **Normalization**: which organizes data for more efficient access.

There are many preprocessing techniques available. Widely used are presented below:

- Common spatial patterns (CSP)
- Independent component analysis (ICA)

3.3.1.1 Common Spatial Patterns (CSP)

The Common Spatial Patterns (CSP) algorithm finds spatial filters that are useful in discriminating different classes of electroencephalogram (EEG) signals such as those corresponding to different types of motor activities. This algorithm involves the estimation of covariance matrices. Using spatial filters, mental activities such as imagined movement can be extracted from the EEG signals. A technique to compute these spatial filters is the common spatial patterns (CSP) algorithm, which has been used successfully for the analysis of imagined movement. The CSP algorithm uses labeled trials to produce a transformation that maximizes the variance for one class while minimizing the variance for the other class. The difference in variance can be used to classify a fragment of EEG signals into one of two classes. While the CSP algorithm is often used in the BCI pipeline, it tends to over fit resulting in a suboptimal performance.[33,34] Several improvements for the CSP have been suggested, but it remains unclear under what circumstances the CSP is more susceptible to over fitting.

The EEG is decomposed into orthogonal signals that can be judged by experts. Afterwards, the signal can be recomposed using only the abnormal signals so that the spatial topography of the abnormal components can be inspected. The CSP algorithm has a tendency to over fit, and a few extensions to the CSP algorithm have been developed in order to improve the generalization performance. A few of these extensions incorporate spatio-spectral filters that include frequency filtering in the CSP algorithm to make it more robust against artifacts. Another extension focuses on scarifying the CSP to prevent over fitting. While these approaches seem to increase the performance it is still unclear what influences the over fitting observed with the CSP algorithm, and therefore it is not known if these changes are adequate.[35]

The CSP algorithm calculates a matrix W with spatial filters with a high variance for the first class and a low variance for the second, and vice versa. It is a $M \times N$ transformation matrix W with the following property:

$$\text{Conv}(W \times 1) = D \text{ and } \text{Conv}(W \times 1) + \text{Conv}(W \times 2) = I \qquad [3.11]$$

where D is a diagonal matrix with elements monotone descending.

I is the identity matrix and $\text{Conv}(X)$ is the covariance matrix of X. N is the number of channels and M is the rank of $\text{Cov}(X)$, and X_i is a matrix with observations in the rows, and EEG channels in the columns for class i. In other words: the transformed channels with a low variance for one class will have a high variance for the other class. This variance can be used for classification. Eq. [3.11] is equivalent to the CSP equations found in Refs 34–36:

$$\text{WConv}(X_1)W^T = D \text{ and } \text{WConv}(X_2)W^T = I - D \qquad [3.12]$$

We can calculate a matrix P using Singular Value Decomposition (SVD) one that will transform the data to have an identity covariance matrix:

$$\text{Conv}(PX) = I \Rightarrow \text{Conv}(X) = (P^T P)^{-1} = U\lambda U^T \qquad [3.13]$$

$$P = \sqrt{\lambda^{-1}U} \qquad [3.14]$$

Where U is an orthogonal matrix, and I is a diagonal matrix. This transformation is equivalent to performing a principal component analysis (PCA) and normalizing the variance to one. When rank $(\text{Cov}(X)) < M$, only the significant eigenvalues and eigenvectors are used to compute P. While $\text{Cov}(PX) = I$, $\text{Cov}(PX_1)$ and $\text{Cov}(PX_2)$ will generally have a covariance matrix that is not completely diagonal. To create a diagonal covariance matrix for $\text{Cov}(WX_1)$ and $\text{Cov}(WX_2)$, we perform an additional SVD after the whitening transform P:

$$\text{Conv}(PX_1) = BDB^T \Rightarrow W = B^T P \qquad [3.15]$$

This definition of W satisfies Eq. [3.11].

3.3.1.2 Independent Component Analysis

Independent Component Analysis (ICA) is a relatively recent method for blind source separation (BSS), which has shown to outperform the classical principal component analysis (PCA) in many applications. In particular, it has been applied for the extraction of ocular artifacts from the EEG, where principal PCA could not separate eye artifacts from brain signals, especially when they have comparable amplitudes.

ICA assumes the existence of n signals that are linear mixtures of m unknown independent source signals. At time instant i, the observed n-dimensional data vector $X(i) = [X_1(i).......X_n(i)]$ is given by the model:[15]

$$X_k(i) = \sum_{j=1}^{m} a_{kj}s_j(i) \quad \text{where } k = 1...n \qquad [3.16]$$

$$X(i) = A^*S(i) \qquad [3.17]$$

where, both the independent source signals $S(i) = [s_1(i)...s_m(i)]$ and the mixing matrix $A = [a_{kj}]$ are unknown. Other conditions for the existence of a solution are (1) $n = m$ (there are at least as many mixtures as the number of independent sources), and (2) up to one source may be Gaussian. Under these assumptions, the ICA seeks a solution of the form:

$$\dot{S} = BX(i) \qquad [3.18]$$

where, B is called the separating matrix.

Recent experiments, as those made by Jung and colleagues,[37] have developed new methods for removing a wide variety of artifacts based on ICA. Over EEG data collected from normal, autistic and brain lesion subjects, ICA could detect, separate, and remove contamination from a wide variety of artifactual sources in EEG records with results comparing favorably to those obtained using regression and others.[38,39] This method presents some advantages compared to other rejection methods, such as:

1. ICA separates EEG signals including artifacts into independent components based on the characteristics of the data, without relying on the availability of one or more "clean" reference channels for each type of artifact. This avoids the problem of mutual contamination between regressing and regressed channels.
2. ICA-based artifact removal can preserve all of the recorded trials, a crucial advantage over rejection-based methods when limited data are available, or when blinks and muscle movements occur too frequently, as in some subject groups.
3. Unlike regression methods, ICA-based artifact removal can preserve data at all scalp channels, including frontal and periocular sites.

3.3.2 Feature Extraction

Feature extraction includes reducing the amount of resources required to describe a large set of data. Feature extraction is the process of defining a set of features, or image characteristics, which will most efficiently or meaningfully represent the information that is important for analysis and classification.

3.3.2.1 Principal Components Analysis

Principal components analysis (PCA) is a widely used mathematical technique to find patterns in data and to represent the data in a way that is more suitable for highlighting the differences between different trials. PCA can be pictured as a rotation of the coordinate axes so that the axes are not along single time points, but along linear combinations of sets of time points which collectively represent a pattern within the signal. PCA rotates the axes in a way that maximizes the variance within the data along the first axis, maintaining the orthogonally of the axes. Mathematically, we represent the data as a matrix X with each column of X being one trial. The task is then to find an orthonormal matrix P such that $Y = PX$ and the covariance matrix for Y is diagonal. The rows of P are then the principal components, ie, an alternative basis for the data, and Y is the data expressed in terms of the alternative basis. If the covariance matrix for Y is diagonal, that means that there is no redundancy between the different dimensions of Y and therefore, one dimension explains as much of the variance in the data as possible; otherwise it would covary with at least one other dimension. The same is true for the second most explanatory dimension, it must explain as much of the leftover variance as possible because otherwise it would covary with one of the remaining dimensions. And so forth for all new dimensions. Conveniently, the amount of variance explained by the ith principal component is equal to the ith diagonal entry of the covariance matrix of Y. Ordering the principal components by the amount of variance they explain provides a way to rank them according to their importance. Finding such a matrix P that satisfies the constraints is not too difficult.[40] In principal components analysis (PCA) one wishes to extract from a set of p variables a reduced set of m components or factors that accounts for most of the variance in the p variables. In other words, we wish to reduce a set of p variables to a set of m underlying super ordinate dimensions.

These underlying factors are inferred from the correlations among the p variables. Each factor is estimated as a weighted sum of the p variables. The ith factor is thus,

$$F_i = W_{i1}X_1 + W_{i2}X_2 + \ldots + W_{ip}X_p \qquad [3.19]$$

One may also express each of the p variables as a linear combination of the m factors,

$$X_j = A_{1j}F_1 + A_{2j}F_2 + \ldots + A_{mj}F_m + U_j \qquad [3.20]$$

where U_j is the variance that is unique to variable j, variance that cannot be explained by any of the common factors.[41,42] The following steps are used for performing PCA:

- Set up the data vectors as the columns of an $(M \times N)$ data matrix X.
- Define the data average vector

$$\mu = \frac{1}{N} \sum_{i=1}^{n} X^k \qquad [3.21]$$

- Compute the covariance matrix XX^T

$$\frac{1}{n-1} \sum_{k=1}^{n} (X^k - \mu)(X^k - \mu)^T \qquad [3.22]$$

- Derive the (eigenvector, eigenvalue) pairs of XX^T and retain them as the set $\{(q^{(i)}, \lambda_j)\}_{j=1}^{r}$ where r is the rank of XX^T. The $q^{(j)}$ eigenvectors are set up as columns in a matrix Q. Their order in Q should correspond to a sort of their eigenvalues in descending order.
- For each $x^{(1)}, x^{(2)}, \ldots, x^{(n)}$, $y^{(k)} = Q^{(T)} x^{(k)}$. The output will be n vectors $y^{(1)}, y^{(2)}, \ldots, y^{(n)}$

3.3.2.2 Mel Frequency Cepstral Coefficients for Speech Feature Extraction

Mel Frequency Cepstral Coefficients (MFCC) technique is robust and dynamic technique for speech feature extraction.[43] Fig. 3.8 shows the complete block diagram of the Mel Frequency Cepstral Coefficients. The Mel-frequency Cepstral Coefficient (MFCC) technique is

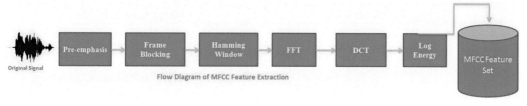

FIGURE 3.8 Block diagram of MFCC.

often used to extract important features of sound file. The MFCC is based on the known variation of the human ear's critical bandwidth frequencies with filters spaced linearly at low frequencies.[44]

In this technique the logarithm of high frequencies is used to capture the important characteristics of speech. From the literature, it is observed that human perception of the frequency contents of sounds for speech signals does not follow a linear scale. Thus, for each tone with an actual frequency, f, measured in Hz, a subjective pitch is measured on a scale called the Mel scale. The Mel-frequency scale is linear frequency spacing below 1000 Hz and a logarithmic spacing above 1000 Hz. As a reference point, the pitch of a 1 kHz tone, 40 dB above the perceptual hearing threshold, is defined as 1000 Mels.

The following formula is used to compute the Mels for a particular frequency:

$$\text{Mel}\,(f) = 2595 \times \log 10\,(1 + f/700). \qquad [3.23]$$

A step by step implementation of the MFCC is shown in Fig. 3.9.[45] In the Pre-emphasis each of the speech samples is sampled at 16,000 Hz for analysis purpose. The sample speech signal was pre-emphasized with filter. In the pre-emphasized the signal is blocked onto the

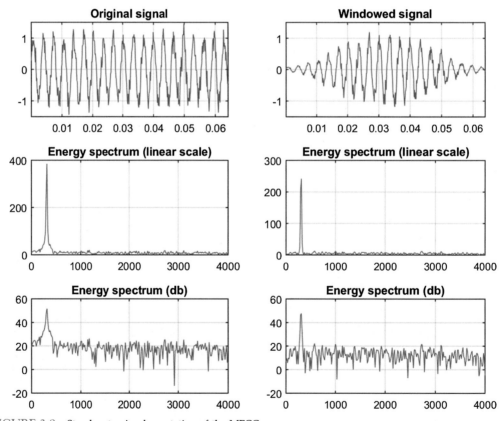

FIGURE 3.9   Step by step implementation of the MFCC.

frame of N sample, with the adjacent frame being separated by M. Finally, the log Mel spectrum was converted into time. The output is called Mel Frequency Cepstrum Coefficients (MFCC). The MFCC is real numbers and it can be converted into time domain using the Discrete Cosine Transform (DCT). The MFCC is used to discriminate the repetitions and prolongations in natural speech.[46] The researcher used MFCC with 12, 13, 26 and 39 variations as original feature and a derivative of it.

3.3.3 Feature Classification

Now a day, the advancements have brought about the exponential development in the feature selection and classification techniques. Both Feature selection and extraction techniques are able to improve learning performance and computational complexity. Classification techniques are identified with a set of categories of observation on the basis of the training data set. The feature classification techniques select the features that are capable of discriminating samples that belong to different classes. Feature classification plays an important role for decision-making tasks in EEG and speech signal analysis by classifying the available information based on some given criteria. There are many possible techniques available for data classification where, linear discriminate analysis, support vector machine and K-NN are robust and dynamic choices for emotion recognition based on speech and EEG signal.[44]

3.3.3.1 *Linear Discriminative Analysis*

Linear Discriminative Analysis (LDA) is a commonly used technique for data classification and dimensionality reduction. It effectively handles the within-class and between-class classification problem. This method maximizes the ratio of between-class variance to the within-class variance in any particular data set thereby guaranteeing maximal classification. The use of Linear Discriminate Analysis for data classification is applied to emotion classification problems in speech and EEG signal. LDA algorithm provides better classification compared to principal components analysis.[48]

This technique doesn't change the location, but only tries to provide more class separability and draw a decision region between the given classes. It has transformed the dataset and test vector are classified by two different approaches.

- Class-dependent LDA approach

  This type of approach includes expanding the ratio of between-class variance to within-class variance. The primary target is to expand this ratio, so that sufficient class classification is obtained. The class-specific type approach involves using two optimizing criteria for transforming the data sets independently.
- Class-independent LDA approach

  This approach involves maximizing the ratio of the overall variance to within-class variance. This approach utilizes stand out advancing the criteria to change the information set and henceforth all information focuses independent of their class character are changed utilizing this change. In this kind of LDA, every class is considered as a different class against every different class.

In the implementation of LDA classification the dimension of data plays an important role. The implementation steps of LDA for two-class problem are explained below.[49]

- Formulate the data sets and the test sets, which are to be classified in the original space. The test and train data become in the matrix form. Assume that the matrix A and B are partitioned into k classes as shown below.

$$A = \begin{bmatrix} a_{11} & a_{12} & a_{13} & a_{14} \\ a_{21} & a_{22} & a_{23} & a_{24} \\ . & . & . & . \\ . & . & . & . \end{bmatrix} \quad B = \begin{bmatrix} b_{11} & b_{12} & b_{13} & b_{14} \\ b_{21} & b_{22} & b_{23} & b_{24} \\ . & . & . & . \\ . & . & . & . \end{bmatrix}$$

- Compute the mean of each data set and mean of the entire data set. Let μ_1 and μ_2 be the means of A and B respectively and μ_3 be mean of entire data, which is obtained by merging A and B, is given by Eq. [3.23].

$$\mu_3 = \rho_1 \times \mu_1 + \rho_2 \times \mu_2 \qquad [3.24]$$

where ρ_1 and ρ_2 are the probabilities of the classes. For the two classes classification value is 0.5.

- The within-class and between-class scatter are used to formulate criteria for class separability. Within-class scatter is the expected covariance of each of the classes. The scatter measures are computed using Eqs. [3.25] and [3.26].

$$S_w = \sum_i \rho_j \times (\text{conv}_j) \qquad [3.25]$$

Therefore for two class classification problem

$$S_w = 0.5 \times \text{conv}_1 + 0.5 \times \text{conv}_2 \qquad [3.26]$$

All the covariance matrices are symmetric. Let conv_1 and conv_2 be the covariance of data A and B respectively. The Covariance matrix is computed using the following Eq. [3.27].

$$S_b = \sum_j (\mu_j - \mu_3) \times (\mu_j - \mu_3)^T \qquad [3.27]$$

The between class scatter is computed using the following Eq. [3.28].

$$\text{conv}_j = (x_j - \mu_j)(x_j - \mu_j)^T \qquad [3.28]$$

S_b is the covariance of the data set, whose members are the mean vectors of each class. As defined earlier, the optimizing criterion in LDA is the ratio of the between-class scatter to the within-class scatter.

- An eigenvector of a transformation represents a 1-D invariant subspace of the vector space. Thus a vector space can be represented in terms of linear combinations of the eigenvectors.

- For any *L*-class problem we would always have $L-1$ non-zero eigenvalues. This is attributed to the constraints on the mean vectors of the classes in Eq. [3.29]. The eigenvectors corresponding to non-zero eigenvalues for the definition of the transformation.
- Once the transformations are completed using the LDA transforms, Euclidean distance or RMS distance is used to classify data points.
- The smallest Euclidean distance among the distances classifies the test vector as belonging to the class.

LDA directions U are determined by Eq. [3.29]. Which can be extended level interpreted as Eq. [3.30]? The objective function implemented in Eq. [3.31];

$$\max_{\mu} T \; \frac{U^T S_b U}{U^T S_w U} \qquad [3.29]$$

$$\min_{\mu} T(U^T S_w U) \; \text{ and } \; \max_{\mu} T(U^T S_b U) \qquad [3.30]$$

$$\max_{\mu} \; \frac{T_r U^T S_b U}{T_r U^T S_w U} \qquad [3.31]$$

LDA has properties like minimizing within-class scatter S_w and/or maximizing between-class scatter S_b as in Eq. [3.30]. It is easy to verify that trace (S_w) measures the closeness of the vectors within the classes, while trace (S_b) measures the separation between classes. Fig. 3.10 represents the graphical representation of LDA classification.

3.3.3.2 *Support Vector Machine*

Support vector machine technique creates a hyper plane in boundless dimensional space, which is classification and regression. A separation is accomplished by the hyper plane that

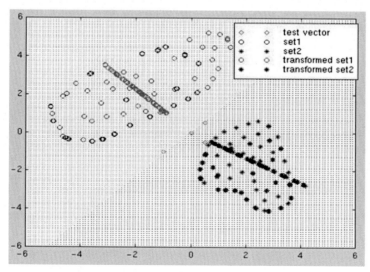

FIGURE 3.10   LDA classification of two class problem.

has the biggest classification for the purpose of nearest training data point of any class. This nearest data point is known as functional margin. The generalization error of the SVM classifier depends on the size of the functional margin.[48]

The SVM training algorithm builds a model on the basis of functional margin; the category of functional margin makes a non-probabilistic binary linear classifier. This technique is a supervised learning model used for linear and non-linear classification. The non-linear classification is performed using kernel based function for mapping input into high dimensional feature space.[51]

3.3.3.2.1 LINEAR CLASSIFICATION

The original linear classification algorithm was proposed by Vapnik in 1963. Support the training data point each belongs to two classes and the objective is to decide which class is responsible for a new data point. In support vector machine a data point is viewed as a ρ dimensional vector and separate data point with a $(\rho - 1)$ dimensional hyper plane is known a linear classification. The steps of linear classification are described below.

- Assume the training data of D with a set of n points of calculating by Eq. [3.32]

$$D = \{(x_i, y_i) | x_i \in \Re^p, y_i \in \{-1,1\}\}_{i=1}^{n} \qquad [3.32]$$

where the y_i is either 1 or -1, indicating the class to which the point x_i belongs. Each x_i is a P-dimensional real vector. We want to find the maximum-margin hyper plane that divides the points having $y_i = 1$ from those having $y_i = -1$
- Any hyper plane can be written as the set of points X satisfying following Eq. [3.33]

$$\mathbf{W} \cdot X - b = 0 \qquad [3.33]$$

where $\cdot$ denotes the dot product and $\mathbf{W}$ denotes the normal vector of hyper plane. The parameter $\frac{b}{\|\mathbf{W}\|}$ determines the offset of the hyper plane from the origin along the normal vector $\mathbf{W}$.
- For maximization distance in point for linearly separable data the margin is set. The set margin hyper plane is described in Eq. [3.34].

$$\mathbf{W} \cdot X - b = 1 \text{ and } \mathbf{W} \cdot X - b = -1 \qquad [3.34]$$

Geometrically, the distance between these two hyper planes is $\frac{2}{\|\mathbf{W}\|}$, so to maximize the distance between the planes we want to minimize $\|\mathbf{W}\|$.
- To prevent the data points to fall into the margin, the following constraint is added: for each i either.

$$\mathbf{W} \cdot X - b \geq 1 \quad \text{For } x_i \text{ of first class}$$
$$\mathbf{W} \cdot X - b \leq 1 \quad \text{For } x_i \text{ of second class}$$

- The final equation is written as Eq. [3.35].

$$y_i(w \cdot x_i - b) \geq 1, \quad \text{for all } 1 \leq i \leq n \qquad [3.35]$$

The extended extension of maximum-margin classifier which provides a solution to the above mentioned problem is given as Eq. [3.36].

$$\text{margin} \equiv \arg \min_{x \in D} d(x) = \arg \min_{x \in D} \frac{X \cdot \mathbf{W} + b}{\sqrt{\sum_{i=1}^{d} w_i^2}} \qquad [3.36]$$

3.3.3.2.2 NON-LINEAR CLASSIFICATION

Non-linear classifier in SVM on the basis of kernel function is proposed by Bernhard E. Boser, Isabelle M. Guyon and Vladimir N. Vapnik. The resulting algorithm and linear classification are formally same, except that every dot product is replaced by a non-linear kernel function. This allows the algorithm to fit the maximum-margin hyper plane in a transformed feature space. The transformation may be non-linear and the transformed space high dimensional; thus though the classifier is a hyper plane in the high-dimensional feature space, it may be non-linear in the original input space.[49]

If the Gaussian radial kernel function used as the corresponding feature space is a Hilbert space for infinite dimensional. This classification shown that higher dimension increases the generalization error, although the amount of feature space is bounded.[50]

- **Kernel Functions**

    The idea of the kernel function is to enable operations to be performed in the input space rather than the potentially high dimensional feature space. Hence the inner product does not need to be evaluated in the feature space. The kernel function plays a critical role in SVM and its performance.

$$K(x, x') = \langle \phi(x), \phi(x') \rangle \qquad [3.37]$$

If K is a symmetric positive definite function, which satisfies Mercer's Conditions,

$$K(x, x') = \sum_{m}^{\infty} a_m \phi_m(x) \phi_m(x'), a_m \geq 0 \qquad [3.38]$$

$$\iint K(x, x') g(x) g(x') dx dx' > 0, g \in L_2 \qquad [3.39]$$

Then the kernel represents a legitimate inner product in feature space. The training set is not linearly separable in an input space. The training set is linearly separable in the feature space.[51,52] Following are the kernel functions used in the non-linear SVM classifier. The performance of classification varies on different kernel function.
- Polynomial (homogeneous) kernel function.

$$k(x_i, x_j) = (x_i \cdot x_j)^d \qquad [3.40]$$

- Polynomial (inhomogeneous) kernel function

$$k(x_i, x_j) = (x_i \cdot x_j + 1)^d \qquad [3.41]$$

- Gaussian radial basis function

$$k(x_i, x_j) = \exp\left(-\gamma \lVert x_i - x_j \rVert^2\right), \quad \text{where } \gamma > 0 \qquad [3.42]$$

- Hyperbolic tangent kernel function

$$k(x_i, x_j) = \tanh(kx_i \cdot x_j + C) \quad \text{Where } k > 0 \text{ and } c < 0 \qquad [3.43]$$

The support vector machine is classified on the basis of number of classes used for the training structure of that class. The following are the extension of SVM.

- **Multiclass SVM**

   Multiclass SVM aims to assign labels to instances by using support vector machines, where the labels are drawn from a finite set of several elements.

- **Transductive support vector machines**

   Transductive support vector machines extend SVMs in that they could also treat partially labeled data in semi-supervised learning by following the principles of transduction.

- **Structured SVM**

   SVMs have been generalized to structured SVMs, where the label space is structured and of possibly infinite size.

This desired hyper plane, which maximizes the margin, also bisects the lines between closest points on convex hull of the two datasets.[21,53] The graphical representation of hyper plane is shown in Fig. 3.11.

Representation of support vector is shown in Fig. 3.12. The solution involves constructing a dual problem and where a Langlier's multiplier α_i is associated.[10] To find w and b such that $\Phi(w) = {}^1/_2 \; |w'||w|$ is minimized; and for all

$$\{(x_i, y_i)\} : y_i(w \times x_i + b) \geq 1 \qquad [3.44]$$

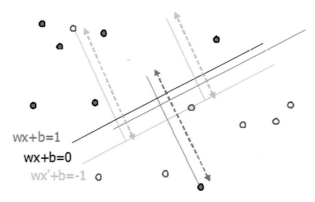

FIGURE 3.11   Representation of Hyper planes.

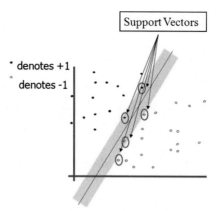

FIGURE 3.12   Representation of support vectors.

Now solving: we get that $w = \Sigma \alpha_i \times x_i$; $b = y_k - \text{w} \times x_k$ for any x_k such that $\alpha_k \neq 0$. Now the classifying function will have the following form:

$$f(x) = \sum \alpha_i y_i x_i \times x + b \qquad [3.45]$$

3.4 CONCLUSION

This chapter explains the technological aspect of rhythm in human brain and speech. The correlation of human brain and speech is explained here. The introduction of brain signal and its functionality are explained. The acoustic phonetic feature is the intermediate between the rhythm of human brain and speech. The focus of this chapter extended towards the acoustic phonetic approach, which is classified as prosodic feature, cepstral measure and voice quality measure based feature. The methodology of speech and brain signal is highlighted here. The necessary mathematical backgrounds associated with relevant signal processing are also discussed.

References

1. What is brain wave [online] http://www.brainworksneurotherapy.com/what-are-brainwaves.
2. Brain wave [online] http://www.transparentcorp.com/products/np/brainwaves.php.
3. Type of wave [Online] http://mentalhealthdaily.com/2014/04/15/5-types-of-brain-waves-frequencies-gamma-beta-alpha-theta-delta/.
4. Gama wave [Online] http://mentalhealthdaily.com/2014/03/12/gamma-brain-waves-40-hz-to-100-hz/.
5. Beta wave [Online] http://mentalhealthdaily.com/2014/04/10/beta-brain-waves-12-hz-to-40-hz/.
6. Alpha wave [Online] http://mentalhealthdaily.com/2014/04/11/alpha-brain-waves-8-hz-to-12-hz/.
7. Theta wave [Online] http://Mentalhealthdaily.Com/2014/04/12/Theta-Brain-Waves-4-Hz-To-8-Hz/.
8. Delta wave [Online] http://Mentalhealthdaily.Com/2014/04/14/Delta-Brain-Waves-0-Hz-To-4-Hz/.
9. Hirose1 K, Minematsu N. *Use of Prosodic Features for Speech Recognition*. 2004.

10. Johnstone T. The Effect of Emotion on Voice Production and Speech Acoustics [thesis]. University of Western Australia & University of Geneva [Online]; 2001. http://Brainimaging.Waisman.Wisc.Edu/~Tjohnstone/Thesis.Pdf.
11. Rong J, Li G, Phoebe Chen YP. Acoustic feature selection for automatic emotion recognition from speech. *Inf Process Manag*. May 2009;45(3):315—328.
12. Bhatlawande SN, Apte SD. Emotion generation using LPC synthesis. *Int J Recent Innovation Trends Comput Commun*. January, 2014;2(1).
13. Schuller B, Rigoll G, Lang M. *Speech Emotion Recognition Combining Acoustic Features and Linguistic Information in a Hybrid Support Vector Machine — Belief Network Architecture*. 2004.
14. Rao KS, Koolagudi SG, Vempada RR. Emotion recognition from speech using global and local prosodic features. *Int J Speech Technol*. June 2013;16(2):143—160.
15. Flaherty MJ, Sidney T. Real time implementation of HMM speech recognition for telecommunication applications. In: *Proceedings of IEEE International Conference on Acoustics, Speech, and Signal Processing, (ICASSP)*. vol. 6. 1994:145—148.
16. Zwicker E, Feldtkeller R. *Das Ohr Als Nachrichtenempfaenger*. Stuttgart: Hirzel Velag; 1967.
17. Meden Y, Yair E, Chazan D. Super resolution pitch determination of speech signals. *IEEE Trans Signal Process*. January 1991;39(1).
18. Gerhard D. *Pitch Extraction and Fundamental Frequency: History and Current Techniques*. November 2003. ISBN:0 7731 0455 0.
19. Eargle JM. *Music, Sound and Technology*. Toronto: Van Nostrand Reinhold; 1995.
20. Handel S. *Listening*. Cambridge: MIT Press; 1989.
21. Lu T-C, Chang CY. A survey of VQ codebook generation. *J Inf Hiding Multimedia Signal Process Ubiquitous Int*. 2010;1(3):190—203.
22. Banerjee A, Merugu S, Dhillon IS, Ghosh J. Clustering with Bregman divergences. *J Mach Learn Res*. 2005;6:1705—1749.
23. Benade AH. *Fundamentals of Musical Acoustics*. London: Oxford University Press; 1976.
24. Lokhande G, Bapat S. Emotion recognition in speech. *Int J Electr Electron Data Commun*. November 2013;1(9). ISSN:2320—2084.
25. Oppenheim A, Schafer AR, Buck J. *Discrete-Time Signame Processing*. 2nd ed. Prentice-Hall; 1999.
26. Johnstone T, Scherer K. The effects of emotions on voice quality. In: *Proceedings of the XIVth Internationl Congress of Phonetic Sciences, San Francisco*. University of Geneva; 1999.
27. Li X, Tao J, Johnson TM, Soltis J, Savage A, Leong KM, et al. *Stress and Emotion Classification Using Jitter and Shimmer Features*. IEEE; 2007. ISBN:1-4244-0728-1/07.
28. Farrús M, Hernando J, Ejarque P, Shimmer J. *Measurements for Speaker Recognition*. 2007.
29. Konar A, Chakrabort A. *Emotion Recognition: a Pattern Analysis Approach*. John Wiley & Sons; December 10, 2014.
30. Alter K, Rank E, Kotz SA, et al. On the relations of semantic and acoustic properties of emotions. In: *Proceedings of the 14th International Conference of Phonetic Sciences (Icphs-99), San Francisco, California*. 1999:2121.
31. Bashashati A, Fatourechi M, Ward RK, Birch GE. Topical review-a survey of signal processing algorithms in brain—computer interfaces based on electrical brain signals. *J Neural Eng*. 2007;4:R32—R57. http://dx.doi.org/10.1088/1741-2560/4/2/R03.
32. Data processing. http://Searchsqlserver.Techtarget.Com/Definition/Data-Preprocessing.
33. Hill NJ, Lal TN, Scholkopf B, et al. Classifying event-related desynchronization in EEC, ECoG, and MEG signals. In: *Toward Brain-Computer Interfacing*. 2007.
34. Lemm S, Blankertz B, Curio G, Muller KR. Spatio-spectral filters for improving the classification of single trial EEG. *Biomed Eng IEEE Trans*. 2005;52(9):1541—1548.
35. Reuderink B, Poel M. *Robustness of the Common Spatial Patterns Algorithm in the BCI-Pipeline*. 2008.
36. Popescu F, Fazli S, Badower Y, Blankertz B, Muller K. Single trial classification of motor imagination using 6 dry EEG electrodes. *PLoS One*. 2007;2(7).
37. Jung TP, Makeig S, Westerfield W, Townsend J, Courchesne E, Sejnowski TJ. Removal of eye activity artifacts from visual event-related potentials in normal and clinical subjects. *Clin Neurophysiol*. 2000;111(10):1745—1758.
38. Jung TP, Humphries C, Lee T-W, Makeig S, Mckeown MJ, Iragui V, et al. Removing electroencephalographic artifacts: comparison between ICA and PCA. *Neural Netw Signal Process*. 1998;VIII:63—72.

39. Schlögl A, Pfurtscheller G. *EOG and ECG minimization based on regression analysis*. Graz, AustriaInstitute for Biomedical Engineering, Department of Medical Informatics, University of Technology; 2001.
40. Shlens J. *Tutorial on Principal Component Analysis*. April 18, 2009.
41. Wuensch KL. *Principal Components Analysis*. 2004.
42. PCA Tutorial CS 898. www.Cs.Odu.Edu/~/Cs495/Lecturenotes/Chapter7/PCA2.Pdf; Viewed 01.01.13.
43. Kesarkar M. *Feature Extraction for Speech Recognition*. Bombay: Indian Institute of Technology; 2003.
44. Patel K, Prasad RK. Speech recognition and verification using MFCC & VQ. *Int J Emerg Sci Eng*. May 2013;1(7). ISSN:2319−6378.
45. Gaikwad S, Gawali B, Mehrotra S. MFCC and TW approach for accent identification. In: *IEEE's International Conferences for Convergence of Technology, Pune, India*. April 5, 2014.
46. Chee LS, Ai OC, Hariharan M, Yaacob S. MFCC based recognition of repetition and prolongations in stuttered speech using k-NN and LDA. In: *Proceedings of 2009 IEEE Student Conferences on Research and Development (Scored 2009), 16−18 Nov.* Serdang, Malaysia: UPM; 2009.
47. Known O-W, Chan K, Lee T-W. Speech feature analysis using variational Bayesian PCA. *IEEE Signal Process Lett*. May 2003;10:137−140.
48 Balakrishnama S, Ganapathiraju A. *Linear Discriminant Analysis − a Brief Tutorial*. Institute for Signal & Information Processing, Department of Electrical & Computer Engineering, Mississipi State University; 2011.
49. Wei Q, Wang Y, et al. Amplitude and phase coupling measures for feature extraction in an EEG − based brain-computer interface. *J Neural Eng*. 2007;4:120−129.
50. Duda R, Hart P. *Pattern Classification and Scene Analysis*. New York: Wiley; 1973.
51. Cristianini N, Taylor JS. *An Introduction to Support Vector Machines and Other Kernel-Based Learning Methods*. Cambridge University Press; 2000.
52. Lewis JP. *Tutorial on SVM*. CGIT Lab, USC; 2004.
53. Furui S. Speaker-independent isolated word recognition using dynamic features of speech spectrum. *IEEE Trans Acoust Speech Signal Process*. 1986;34(1):52−59.

4

Time and Frequency Analysis

4.1 INTRODUCTION

The time domain is the analysis of mathematical functions, physical signals, or time series of data with respect to time. In the time domain, the signal or function's value is known for all real numbers in the case of continuous time, or at various separate instants in the case of discrete time. There are various tools used to acquire and display these signals. Two tools to acquire brain and speech signals are described in other chapters of the book. In this chapter we describe mathematical techniques to analyze time-dependent signals by transforming them into frequency or some other domain. Time-dependent signals show how the values of a signal changes with time, whereas a frequency domain graph shows the

Introduction to EEG- and Speech-Based Emotion Recognition
http://dx.doi.org/10.1016/B978-0-12-804490-2.00004-X

81

variation of power with respect to frequency. Fourier transformation, window-based Fourier transformation, and wavelet transformation are described in detail, along with their strengths and limitations. Various relevant examples are also given to illustrate their significance.

4.2 FOURIER TRANSFORMATION

As mentioned in earlier chapters, electroencephalogram (EEG) and speech signals are both acquired in the time domain. A time-dependent signal gives a clear visualization, such as periodicity and abrupt changes. Time-dependent signals may be transformed into another domain to see other characteristics in the signals. Frequency domain representation is the most commonly used and the most powerful tool to see clearly periodicity characteristics in the signal. The advantage of frequency domain representation is being able to understand underlying physical phenomena. Frequency-time representation analysis, developed by Jean Baptiste Fourier (1768–1830), has innumerable applications in mathematics, physics, and natural sciences. Furthermore, Fourier transformation is computationally very attractive, since it can be calculated by using an extremely efficient algorithm called the Fast Fourier Transform (FFT).[1]

4.2.1 Theoretical Background

The Fourier transformation of a continuous time-dependent signal $x(t)$ may be considered as a linear superposition of sines and cosines characterized by their frequency f and given by Eqs. [4.1] and [4.2] as follows:

$$x(t) = \int_{-\infty}^{+\infty} X(f)e^{i2\pi ft} df \qquad [4.1]$$

$$X(f) = \int_{-\infty}^{+\infty} x(t)e^{-i2\pi ft} dt \qquad [4.2]$$

Eq. [4.2] may be considered as the frequency representation of the time-dependent signal $x(t)$, whereas Eq. [4.1] is a time representation of a frequency-dependent signal $X(f)$ which is complex in nature.

Eq. [4.2] may also be considered as an inner product of the signal $x(t)$ with complex sinusoidal orthogonal basis (mother) functions, $\exp(-i2\pi ft)$, expressed as:

$$X(f) = < x(t), e^{-i2\pi ft} > \qquad [4.3]$$

Its inverse transformation is given by Eq. [4.1], and since the basis functions $\exp(-i2\pi ft)$ are orthogonal, the Fourier transformation is nonredundant and unique.

The signal $x(n)$ may be considered as N discrete values, sampled at a constant interval of time Δ, with its value as x_i at time $t_i = t_0 + i\,\Delta(i = 0,N-1)$:

$$x(n) = \{x_0, x_1, ..., x_{N-1}\} = \{x_j\} \qquad [4.4]$$

The discrete Fourier transformation of this signal is defined as:

$$X(k) = \sum_{n=0}^{N-1} x(n)e^{-i2\pi kn/N} \quad k = 0, \dots, N-1 \tag{4.5}$$

and its inverse as:

$$x(n) = \frac{1}{N} \sum_{k=0}^{N-1} X(k)e^{i2\pi kn/N} \tag{4.6}$$

Since we are considering real signals, the following relation holds: $X(k) = X^*(N-k)$, where X^* is a complex conjugate of X, and the discrete frequencies are defined as:

$$f_k = \frac{k}{N\Delta} \tag{4.7}$$

Note that the discrete Fourier transformation gives $N/2$ independent complex coefficients, thus giving a total of N values as in the original signal and therefore being nonredundant. The frequency resolution will be:

$$\Delta f = \frac{1}{N\Delta} \tag{4.8}$$

4.2.2 Aliasing

The frequency $f_N = 1/2\Delta$ corresponding to $k = N/2$ in Eq. [4.7] is called the Nyquist frequency, and is the highest frequency that can be detected in a sampling period Δ.

If the signal $x(n)$ has frequencies above the Nyquist frequency, these will be processed just as though they are in the range $f_k < f_N$, thus giving a spurious effect called aliasing.[2,3] The greater this excess is, the greater the errors and the less adequate is the sampling rate Δ for representing the signal. From the complex coefficients of Eq. [4.5], the periodogram can be obtained as:

$$I_{xx}(k) = |X(k)|^2 = X(k) \cdot X^*(k) \tag{4.9}$$

where * denotes a complex conjugation. The sample cross-spectrum can be similarly defined by making the product of Eq. [4.9] between two time series $x(n)$ and $y(n)$ as follows:

$$I_{xy}(k) = X(k) \cdot Y^*(k) \tag{4.10}$$

where $X(k)$ and $Y(k)$ are the Fourier transformations of $x(t)$ and $y(t)$ respectively. The sample cross-spectrum gives a measure of the linear correlation between two signals for the different frequencies f_k, defined as in Eq. [4.7]. Since it is a complex measure, it can be described by an amplitude and a phase. A useful measure of the amplitude is obtained with its square value, normalized in the following way:

$$\Gamma^2_{xy}(k) = \frac{|I_{xy}(k)|^2}{I_{xy}(k) \cdot I_{yy}(k)} \tag{4.11}$$

Eq. [4.11] is known as the squared coherence function, and it will give values tending to one for highly linearly correlated signals and to zero for noncorrelated signals. The counterpart of coherence is the phase function, defined as:

$$\Phi = \arctan \frac{-\mathbf{I}(I_{xy}(k))}{\mathbf{R}(I_{xy}(k))} \qquad [4.12]$$

where $\mathbf{I}$ means the imaginary part and $\mathbf{R}$ the real one. It should be noted that the phase is meaningful only when the coherence is significant. If this is the case, Φ gives a measure of the time delay between the two signals according to the following formula[4]

$$t = \frac{\Phi}{2\pi f_k} \qquad [4.13]$$

where Φ is the phase difference in degrees at a frequency f_k (defined in Eq. [4.7]).

4.3 GABOR TRANSFORMATION (SHORT-TIME FOURIER TRANSFORMATION)[5-7]

The main disadvantage of the Fourier transformation technique is that it does not provide information regarding the time evolution of the frequencies. If some alteration occurs at some boundary, the whole Fourier spectrum will get changed. Thus the technique is applicable only to stationary waves. Fourier transformation also cannot define the instantaneous frequency because it integrates over the whole time, thus giving a broad frequency spectrum.

The problems associated with Fourier transformation can partially be resolved by using the Gabor transformation, also known as short-time Fourier transformation. The concept of Gabor transformation is to break the signal into small time segments using an appropriate sliding-window function, and then apply a Fourier transformation to the successive sliding-window segments. Thus the evolution of the frequencies can be followed, and the stationary requirement is partially satisfied by considering the signals to be stationary in the order of the window length.

4.3.1 Theoretical Considerations

Gabor transformation of a time-dependent signal $x(t)$ is very similar to Fourier transformation, except it is modulated by an appropriate sliding window of width D. It is expressed as:

$$\mathscr{G}_D(f,t) = \int_{-\infty}^{\infty} x(t')g_D^*(t'-t)e^{-i2\pi ft'}\,dt' \qquad [4.14]$$

where $g_D(t'-t)$ is the window function of width D centered in t. * represents the complex conjugation. Analogous with Fourier transformation, Gabor transformation can be considered as an inner product between the signal and the complex sinusoidal functions $e^{-i2\pi ft'}$ modulated by the window $g_D(t)$. Therefore, Eq. [4.14] may also be expressed as:

$$\mathscr{G}_D(f,t) = \; <x(t'), g_D(t'-t)e^{-i2\pi ft'}> \qquad [4.15]$$

The property of the window function should be such that it peaks around t and falls off rapidly, thus emphasizing the signal at time t and suppressing it for distant times. Several window functions have been used to achieve this, and one popular choice is a Gaussian function, as follows:[8]

$$g_\alpha(t) = \left(\frac{\alpha}{\pi}\right)^{1/4} e^{\frac{-\alpha}{2}t^2}$$

[4.16]

where α is a decay parameter which determines the rate at which the function asymptotically approaches zero. The Gaussian function can be truncated to have a length D, by assuming that in the border their values are nearly zero due to use of a reasonable appropriate value of α. Thus the Gabor transformation can be explicitly defined as a function of the parameter α:

$$\mathscr{G}_D(f,t) \rightarrow \mathscr{G}_D^\alpha(f,t)$$

[4.17]

It is possible to derive the inverse of the Gabor transformation as follows:

$$x(t) = \frac{1}{\|g_D\|} \int_{-\infty}^{\infty} \int_{-\infty}^{\infty} \mathscr{G}_D(f,t') \cdot g_D(t-t') e^{i2\pi ft} df\, dt'$$

[4.18]

where $\|g_D\| = \int_{-\infty}^{\infty} \left| g_D(t') \right|^2 dt'$.

Gabor transformation is highly redundant because it gives a time-frequency map from every time value of the original signal. To decrease redundancy, a sampled Gabor transformation can be defined by taking discrete values of time and frequency:

$$\mathscr{G}_D(f,t) \rightarrow \mathscr{G}_D(mF, nT)$$

[4.19]

where F and T represent the frequency and time sampling steps. Smaller F means a larger window, and smaller T means more overlapping between successive windows.

The spectrum of the signal may be defined as:

$$I(f,t) = \left| \mathscr{G}_D(f,t) \right|^2 = \mathscr{G}_D^*(f,t) \cdot \mathscr{G}_D(f,t)$$

[4.20]

Spectrograms of the signal can be obtained by sliding the window and getting a time-frequency representation. The band power spectral intensity can be obtained as follows:

$$I^{(i)}(t) = \int_{f_{min}^{(i)}}^{f_{max}^{(i)}} I(f,t) df \quad i = \delta, \theta, \alpha, \ldots$$

[4.21]

where $(f_{min}^{(i)}, f_{max}^{(i)})$ are the frequency limits of band i. Examples of these bands with respect to EEG signals are illustrated in Chapter 3.

The total power spectral density may be obtained by summing the power related to all bands, as follows:

$$I_T(t) = \sum_i I^{(i)}(t) \quad i = \delta, \theta, \alpha, \ldots$$

[4.22]

The band relative intensity ratio for the ith band may be defined as:

$$\text{RIR}^{(i)}(t) = \frac{I^{(i)}(t)}{I_T(t)} \times 100 \qquad [4.23]$$

For further quantitative analysis, the band mean weight frequency may be defined as:

$$<f^{(i)}(t) \geq \left[\int_{f^{(i)}_{\min}}^{f^{(i)}_{\max}} I(f,t)f\,df \right] \Big/ I^{(i)}(t) \qquad [4.24]$$

and the band maximum peak frequency $f_{M(i)}$ of the ith band as the frequency value for which $I(f,t)$ is maximum in the interval $(f^{(i)}_{\min}, f^{(i)}_{\max})$ at time t:

$$I(f_M, t) > I(f, t) \quad \forall \ f \neq f_M \in \left(f^{(i)}_{\min}, f^{(i)}_{\max} \right) \qquad [4.25]$$

4.3.2 Limitations of Gabor Transformation[5,6,9]

One critical limitation of the window-based approach is related to time and frequency resolution. According to the uncertainty principle, sharp localizations in time and frequency are mutually exclusive because a frequency cannot be determined instantaneously. This means if the window is too narrow, the frequency resolution will be poor, and if the window is too wide, the time localization will not be so precise.

If σ_t is the uncertainty in time and σ_f is corresponding uncertainty in frequency, the uncertainty principle can be expressed as follows:

$$\sigma_t \cdot \sigma_f \geq \frac{1}{4\pi} \qquad [4.26]$$

Here it is assumed that the signals are normalized. The limitation becomes serious when the signal has transient components localized in time.

4.4 SHORT-TIME FOURIER TRANSFORMATION

The short-time Fourier transformation (STFT) function is simply Fourier transformation operating on a small section of the data. After the transformation is complete on one section of the data, the next selection is transformed, and the output "stacked" next to the previous transformation output. This method is very similar to Gabor transformation, as mentioned above; the only difference is the types of window used. Popular types of window functions are rectangular, Hamming, Hanning, and Blackman-Tukey. All these windows have similar properties as those used with Gabor transformation.

4.4.1 Window Size for Short-Term Spectral Analysis[10,11]

The window size depends on the type of time-varying signals. We can minimize the effect of window size by using a proper size of window. For example, in the case of speech-related signals, the window length may be selected as 10–30 m. By selecting the proper size, the spectral information may be affected to a minimal extent. If the window size is too small, the window effect may be too severe. Alternatively, if the window is too large then even though the windowing effect is negligible compared to the 10–30 m case, we cannot use such a long window due to the nonstationary nature of speech.[10]

In case of short-term spectral analysis, we consider speech in segments of 10–30 m. For a given frame size, the nature of spectral information may vary slightly depending on the type of window, which is essentially a finite-duration function used for selecting a particular segment of speech. However, the nature of the window function varies the spectral information. Fig. 4.1 shows the rectangular, Hamming, and Hanning window functions in the time and frequency domains. The width of main lose in the frequency domain is less for the rectangular window compared to the other two window functions. As a result the resolution offered by the rectangular window function is better. However, the peak-to-side lobe ratio of the rectangular window is significantly poor compared to the other two windows. This results in relatively more spectral leakage in the rectangular window, which is not desirable. Thus from a resolution point of view the rectangular window is preferable and from a spectral leakage point of view the other two window functions are preferable. The effect of spectral leakage is severe, and hence in most speech analysis applications either a Hamming or a Hanning window is employed.

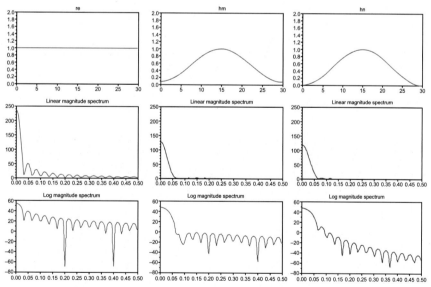

FIGURE 4.1   Rectangular, Hamming, and Hanning windows and their spectra.

4.5 WAVELET TRANSFORMATION

As explained in earlier sections, due to the uncertainty principle, the modified Fourier transformation using a uniform window limits resolutions in time and frequency measurements, as per Eq. [4.26]. The above-mentioned techniques are not suitable for analyzing signals involving different ranges of frequencies. Data involving slow processes require wide windows, and for data with fast transients a narrow window is more suitable.

Grossmann and Morlet[12] introduced wavelet transformation to overcome this problem. The main advantage of wavelets is that they have varying window size, being wide for slow frequencies and narrow for fast ones. This leads to optimal time-frequency resolution in all frequency ranges.[6,12,13,14] Furthermore, owing to the fact that windows are adapted to the transients of each scale, wavelets do not require stationarity.

4.5.1 Theoretical Background

4.5.1.1 *Continuous Wavelet Transformation*

A wavelet family $\psi_{a,b}(t)$ is a set of elemental functions generated by dilations and translations of a unique mother wavelet (t):

$$\psi_{a,b}(t) = |a|^{-1/2}\psi\left(\frac{t-b}{a}\right) \tag{4.27}$$

where a and b are the scale and translation parameters. Both are real numbers, and a is nonzero. As the scale parameter a increases, the wavelet becomes narrower; and by varying translation parameter b, the mother wavelet is displayed in time.

The continuous wavelet transformation of a real-time signal $X(t)$ is defined as the correlation between the signal and the wavelet functions $\psi_{a,b}$, expressed as:

$$(W_\psi X)(a,b) = \left|a\right|^{-1/2} \int_{-\infty}^{\infty} X(t)\psi^*\left(\frac{t-b}{a}\right)dt = <X(t), \psi_{a,b}> \tag{4.28}$$

where * denotes complex conjugation. Then a different correlation of $<X(t),\psi_{a,b}>$ indicates how precisely the wavelet function locally fits the signal at every scale a. Since the correlation is made with different scales of a single function, instead of with complex sinusoids characterized by their frequencies, wavelets give a time-scale representation.

4.5.1.2 *Dyadic Wavelet Transformation*

Continuous wavelet transformation maps a signal of one independent variable, t, on to a function of two independent variables, a and b. This procedure is redundant and not efficient for algorithm implementation. In consequence, it is more practical to define the wavelet transformation only at discrete scale a and discrete time b. One way to achieve this is by choosing the discrete set of parameters $\{a_j = 2^j\ b_{j,k} = 2^j k\}$, with $j, k \in Z$. Replacing these in Eq. [4.27], we obtain the discrete wavelet family:

$$\psi_{j,k}(t) = 2^{-j/2}\psi\left(2^{-j}t - k\right) \quad j,k \in \mathcal{Z} \tag{4.29}$$

that forms a basis of the Hilbert space, and whose correlation with the signal is called dyadic wavelet transformation.

4.5.1.3 Multiresolution Analysis

High-frequency components of the signal will be matched with contracted versions of the wavelet functions, while dilated versions will match low-frequency oscillations. Thus it is possible to get details of the signal at different scale levels by correlating the signal with wavelet functions of different sizes. A hierarchical scheme known as multiresolution analysis is used to organize the information given by the dyadic wavelet transformation.[6,13]

Consider W_j belongs to the subspaces of $\mathscr{L}^2$ generated by the wavelet $\psi_{j,k}$ for each level j, the space $\mathscr{L}^2$ can be decomposed as a direct sum of the subspace W_j:

$$\mathscr{L}^2 = \sum_{j \in \mathscr{Z}} W_j \qquad [4.30]$$

The closed subspaces may be defined as:

$$V_j = W_{j+1} \oplus W_{j+2} \ldots \quad j \oplus \mathscr{Z} \qquad [4.31]$$

The subspaces V_j are a multiresolution approximation of $\mathscr{L}^2$, and are generated by scaling and translations of a single function $\varphi_{j,k}$, called the scaling function. For the subspace V_j the orthogonal complementary subspaces W_j can be obtained as:

$$V_{j-1} = V_j \oplus W_j \quad j \in \mathscr{Z} \qquad [4.32]$$

Let us suppose we have a discrete signal $X(n)$, which will denote x_0, with finite energy and without loss of generality; let us also suppose that the sampling rate is $\Delta t = 1$. Then we can successively decompose it with a recursive scheme:

$$x_{j-1}(n) = x_j \oplus r_j(n) \qquad [4.33]$$

where the term $x_j(n)$ belongs to V_j and gives the coarser representation of the signal, and $r_j(n)$ belongs to W_j and gives the details for each scale $j = 0, 1, \ldots, N$. Then, for any resolution level $N > 0$, we can write the decomposition of the signal as:

$$X(n) = \sum_k x_N(k)\phi(2^{-N}n - k) + \sum_{j=1}^{N} \sum_k C_j(k)\psi_{j,k}(n) \qquad [4.34]$$

where $\phi(.)$ is the scaling function, $C_j(k)$ are the wavelet coefficients, and the sequence $\{x_N(k)\}$ represents the coarser signal at resolution level N. The second term is the wavelet expansion. The wavelet coefficients $C_j(k)$ can be interpreted as the local residual errors between successive signal approximations at scale $j-1$ and j, and:

$$r_j(n) = \sum_k C_j(k)\psi_{j,k}(n) \qquad [4.35]$$

is the detail signal at scale j.

The selection of a suitable mother function to be compared with the signal is very important. As mentioned above, not every function can be used as a wavelet. One criterion for choosing the wavelet function is that it should have similar patterns to the original signal. In this respect, B-Spline functions are suitable for decomposing.

4.5.1.4 Discrete Wavelet (Haar) Transformation

Discrete wavelet Haar transformation uses a different basis than STFT. STFT uses complex sinusoids with increasing frequency, which are shaped by the window function. Wavelet transformations, on the other hand, maintain the same number of oscillations within the window, but compress or dilate the window to adjust the frequency. The method has other properties, such as that the function must always be band pass. A wide variety of basis functions are available. We used the most basic: the Haar wavelet.

4.5.1.5 The Morlet Wavelet

The continuous wave form was introduced earlier. The wavelet function is analogous to the windowing function of the STFT and scale is analogous to frequency. The wavelet function must be square integrable and band pass (have no energy at zero frequency). We used a real Morlet wavelet, which holds the above properties and has the following form:

$$w(t) = \frac{1}{K\sigma}\, e^{-(\sigma t)^2}\cos(2\pi f_0\, t) \qquad [4.36]$$

where sigma is the approximate bandwidth and f_0 is the center frequency. Fig. 4.2 shows examples of the Morlet wavelet function at three different scales, along with the corresponding frequency domain information.

Note that frequency resolution is proportional to bandwidth, so it will decrease at higher frequencies and increase at lower frequencies. Accordingly, we get higher time resolution at

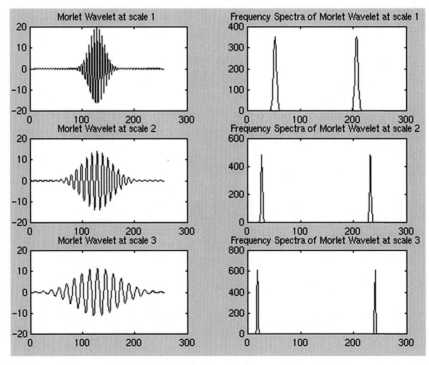

FIGURE 4.2   The Morlet wavelet at different scales.

higher frequencies and lower time resolution at lower frequencies. This is not the case in STFT, where the frequency resolution is the same over all frequencies. Finally, we implement continuous wavelet transformation by sampling at $t = n/s$.

4.6 TIME DOMAIN VERSUS FREQUENCY DOMAIN ANALYSIS

The time domain and the frequency domain are two modes used to analyze data. Both time domain analysis and frequency domain analysis are widely used in electronics, acoustics, telecommunications, and many other fields.

- Frequency domain analysis is used in conditions where processes such as filtering, amplifying, and mixing are required.
- Time domain analysis gives the behavior of the signal over time. This allows predictions and regression models for the signal.
- Frequency domain analysis is very useful in creating desired wave patterns, such as binary bit patterns of a computer.
- Time domain analysis is used to understand data sent in such bit patterns over time.

4.7 EXAMPLES

Basic theoretical concepts used in time-frequency analysis have been used extensively in various fields of medicine and engineering. Fig. 4.3 shows a typical example of a speech signal which is transformed into the frequency domain using a Hamming window of

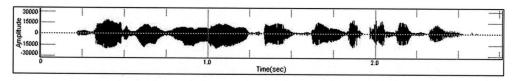

Waveform for the Sentence :"There was no answer from the other side"

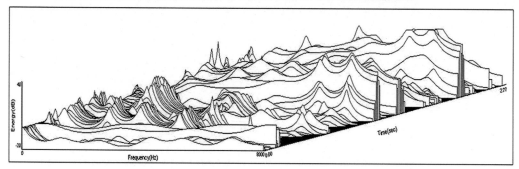

FIGURE 4.3   Speech signal in time domain (above) and representation in frequency domain (below).

250 ms. The frequency spectrum shows time-dependent peaks to identify the characteristics of spoken speech.[15]

Fig. 4.4 shows the analysis as obtained by Fourier, Gabor, and wavelet transformations. In this example, Fourier transformation is obtained by correlating the original signal with complex sinusoids of different frequencies (top). In the Gabor transformation, the signal is correlated with modulated sinusoidal functions that slide upon the time axis, thus giving a time-frequency representation (middle). Wavelets give an alternative time-scale representation, but due to their varying window size a better resolution for each scale is achieved (bottom). Furthermore, the function to be correlated with the original signal can be chosen depending on the application (eg, in the graph quadratic B-Splines wavelets are shown).[16]

In Fig. 4.5 the signal is decomposed in scale levels, each representing the activity in different frequency bands. The wavelet coefficients show how closely the signal matches locally the different dilated versions of the wavelet mother function (in this case a quadratic B-Spline). Furthermore, by applying the inverse transformation, the signal can be reconstructed from the wavelet coefficients for each scale level.[16]

Fig. 4.6 shows an EEG signal acquired in a thought experiment.[17] In this case the subject was trained to think about the digit "0." The Gabor transformation of the signal is shown in Fig. 4.7. A part of the signal was analyzed through continuous wavelet transformation, and the results are shown in Figs. 4.8 and 4.9.

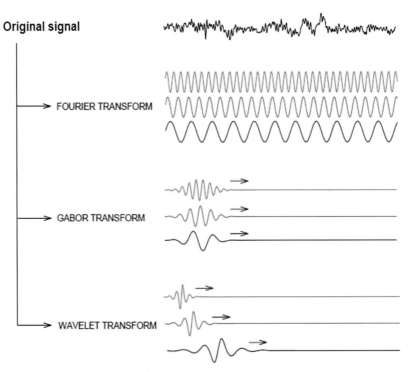

FIGURE 4.4   Illustration of mother functions in Fourier, Gabor, and wavelet transformations.

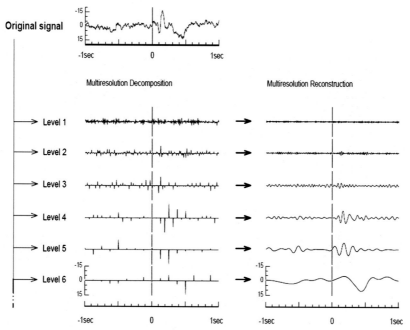

FIGURE 4.5   Multiresolution decomposition method.

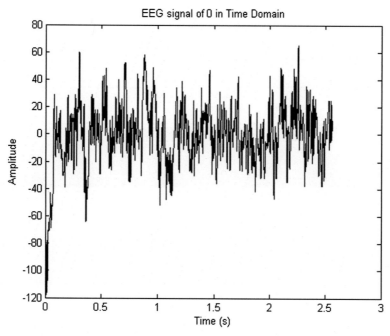

FIGURE 4.6   A typical EEG signal in a thought experiment.

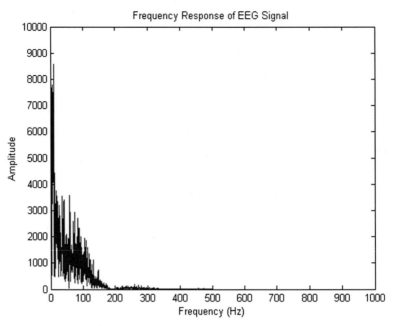

FIGURE 4.7   Fourier transformation of the signal given in Fig. 4.6.

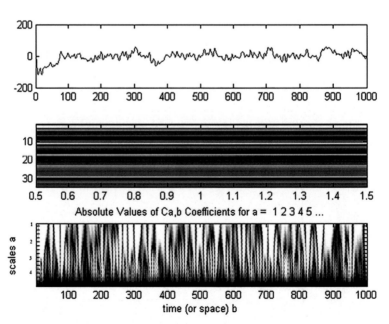

FIGURE 4.8   Continuous wavelet transformation of the signal given in Fig. 4.6.

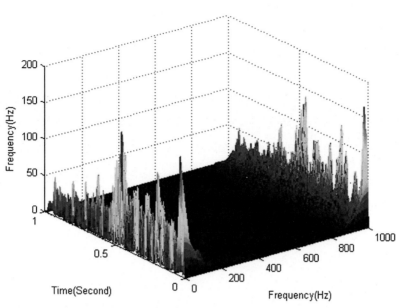

FIGURE 4.9   The three-dimensional representation of the wavelet for the signal.

4.8 CONCLUSION

Time-varying signals may be transformed to the frequency domain by using various transformations. Fourier transformation is suitable if the signal is stationary and frequency components do not change with time. But real-world signals like brain and speech signals change with time. These signals can be analyzed using sliding-window-based Fourier transformation methods by choosing an appropriate window size and overlapping successive sliding windows. The uncertainty principle limits resolutions related to time and frequency in a constant-size window. Wavelet transformation is suitable to analyze such signals. This is illustrated by many examples related to signals in the real world.

References

1. Cooley WJ, Tukey JW. An algorithm for the machine calculation of complex Fourier series. *Math Comput.* 1965:297–301.
2. Weaver HJ. *Theory of Discrete and Continous Fourier Analysis.* Wiley-Interscience; 1989.
3. Jenkins GM, Watts D. *Spectral Analysis and Applications.* San Fracisco: Holden-Day; 1968.
4. Brazier MAN. Speed of seizure discharges in epilepsy: anatomical and electrophysiological considerations. *Exp Neurol.* 1972;36:263–272.
5. Chui C. *An Introduction to Wavelets.* San Diego: Academic Press; 1992.
6. Cohen L. *Time Frequency Analysis.* Prentice-Hall; 1965.
7. Qian S, Chan D. *Joint Time-Frequency Analysis: Methods and Applications.* NJ: Printice Hall; 1996.
8. Gabor D. Theory of communication. *J Inst Elec Eng.* 1946;93:429–459.
9. Kaiser G. *A Friendly Guide to Wavelets.* Boston: Birkhaeuser; 1994.

10. Harris FJ. On the use of windows for Harmonic analysis with the discrete Fourier transform. *Proc IEEE*. 1978;66(1):51—83.
11. Toraichi K, Kamada M, Itahashi S, Mori R. Window functions represented by B-spline functions. *IEEE Trans Acoust Speech Signal Process*. 1989;37:145.
12. Grossmann, Morlet. Decomposition of Hardy functions into square integrable wavelets of constant shape. *SIAM J Math Anal*. 1984;15:723—736.
13. Mallat SA. A theory for multiresolution signal decomposition: the wavelet representation. *IEEE Trans Pattern Anal Mach Intell*. 1989;2(7):674—693.
14. Strang G, Nguyen T. *Wavelets and Filter Banks*. Wellesley: Wellesley-Cambridge Press; 1996.
15. Gawali BW. unpublished work.
16. Quiroga RQ. *Quantitative Analysis of EEG Signals: Time-Frequency Methods and Chaos Theory* [Ph.D. thesis]. Lübeck: Medical University; 1998.
17. Deore R, Gawai G, Mehrotra S. *Digit Recognition System Using EEG Signal*. Springer International Publishing; 2015:375—416.

CHAPTER

5

Emotion Recognition

5.1 INTRODUCTION

Emotions may be considered to be a feeling that results in physical and psychological changes that control our behavior. Progress in emotion recognition has significantly advanced over the past two decades, with the contribution of many disciplinary fields like psychology, neuroscience, endocrinology, medicine, sociology, and even computer science.

For recognition of emotions, brain activity is essential, involving motivation, perceptual experience, knowledge, cognition, creativity, attention, learning, and decision-making. Basically, there are two broad classes of recognition of emotions with three different modalities.[1]

- Unimodal: recognition of emotions using only one modality as input to the system.
- Bimodal: the recognition system includes two modalities as input to the system.
- Multimodal: includes more than two modalities for recognition of emotions.

5.2 MODALITIES FOR EMOTION RECOGNITION SYSTEMS

The term modality implies the type of expression. The psychology of perception suggests that the cognitive system uses sensory and sign modalities to convey some meaning.

Introduction to EEG- and Speech-Based Emotion Recognition
http://dx.doi.org/10.1016/B978-0-12-804490-2.00005-1

Sensory modalities can include any form of senses—visual, auditory, tactile, etc. A list of sign types would include writing, symbol, index, image, map, graph, and diagram.

Thus technologically the modality refers to a certain type of information and/or the representation format in which information is stored. Modalities can be grouped in three different categories, as represented in Fig. 5.1.[2]

5.2.1 Physiological

Physiology is the scientific study of the normal function in living systems, and aims to understand the function of living things. Human physiology studies the interconnection of muscles and organs as well as their interaction.

5.2.1.1 Facial Expression

The face plays a significant role in human communication. It acts as a "window" to human personality, emotions, thoughts, and ideas. Psychological research conducted by Mehrabian[3] established the importance of the face, proving that it contributes around 55 percent in recognition of information, including the nonverbal part which is the most informative channel in social communication. The verbal part contributes about 7 percent of the message, while 34 percent of the message is contributed through acoustic properties (vocal) such as tone, energy of speech and 55 percent through facial expression. This makes the face a powerful entity in recognition of emotion in many areas, such as psychology, behavioral science, medicine, and computer science.[4] It not only distinguishes a person's characteristics and identity, but also carries large amount of information about the person's emotional characteristics.[5-6] The face is considered not only as a reflection of a person's identity, but also reveals a large amount of emotional attributes.[6]

In recent years there has been expanding interest in all aspects of interaction between humans and computers, especially in the area of emotion recognition by observing facial expressions.[7-8] Facial expression recognition has a tremendous scope of applications in fields

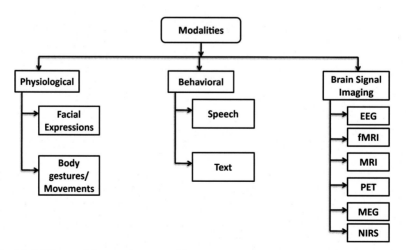

FIGURE 5.1   Modalities used for emotion recognition systems.

such as developing friendly human—machine interfaces to give communication analogous to human communication, behavioral science, clinical studies, psychological treatment, video conferencing, and many more.[8]

5.2.1.1.1 FEATURES FOR FACIAL EXPRESSIONS

Feature extraction is the process of defining a set of features, or image characteristics, which will most efficiently or meaningfully represent the information that is important for analysis and classification. Face expression is an important area of research, dealing with recognition of emotions through the face. The various features corresponding to different emotions are described in Table 5.1.

5.2.1.1.2 FACIAL ACTION CODING SYSTEM

The Facial Action Coding System (FACS) is a system to develop taxonomies of human facial movements by their appearance on the face, based on a system originally developed by the Swedish anatomist Carl-Herman Hjortsjö.[9] It was later adapted by Paul Ekman and Wallace V. Friesen, and published in 1978.[10] Ekman, Friesen, and Joseph C. Hager published a significant update to FACS in 2002. Movements of individual facial muscles are encoded by FACS from slight, different, or instant changes in facial appearance.[11]

FACS is an index of facial expressions, but does not actually provide any biomechanical information about the degree of muscle activation. The primary goal in developing FACS was to achieve a comprehensive system which could describe all possible visually distinguishable facial movements, since every facial movement is the result of muscular action. Each facial action is described in sufficient detail and exactness, and an attempt is made to apply that description to the flow of facial behavior.

Using FACS, human coders can manually code nearly any anatomically possible facial expression, deconstructing it into the specific action units (AUs) and their temporal segments that produced the expression. AUs are the underlying activities of single muscles or groups of muscles. FACS AUs are based on what the muscles allow the face to do, and are associated with one or more facial muscles. There are 44 different AUs in FACS, related to the contraction of either a specific facial muscle or a set of facial muscles.

FACS is designed to be self-instructional. Users can learn the technique from a number of sources, including manuals and workshops, and obtain certification through testing.[11]

FACS is a common standard for systematic categorization of the physical expression of emotions. Recently it has been turned into a computerized automated system that detects faces in videos, extracts their geometrical features, and then produces temporal profiles of each facial movement. FACS is a key system in determining facial feature extraction.

Much research work has used FACS as a framework for classification of emotions. Paul Ekman studied the changes of muscular contractions and used them to identify emotions. Previous studies had traditionally taken two approaches to emotion classification: judgment based and sign based.[12]

The judgment-based approach develops the categories of emotion in advance; for example categorizing the emotions in the traditional six universal emotions. The sign-based approach uses a FACS system, ie, encoding AUs to categorize an expression based on its characteristics. The approach assigns an emotional value to a facial expression using a combination of the key AUs that create the expression. A neural network is used to recognize AUs from the coordinates of facial features like lip corners or the curve of eyebrows.[13]

TABLE 5.1   Features Used in Facial Action Coding System Describing Different Emotional States

Component of face	Emotions						
	Happy	Sad	Neutral	Surprise	Fear	Anger	Disgust
Eyes	Lower eyelid shows wrinkles below it Wrinkles around outer corners of eyes	Inner corners of eyebrows are drawn up	No expression	Eyelids opened wide	Upper eyelid is raised and lower eyelid is drawn up	No expression	No expression
Eyebrows	No expression	Upper lid inner corner is raised	No expression	Brows raised Skin below brow stretched, not wrinkled	Brows raised and drawn together	Brows lowered and drawn together Lines appear between brows Lower lid tense/may be raised Upper lid tense/lowered due to brows' action	Brows lowered
Lips	Lip endings are placed back and up mouth parted/not with teeth exposed/ not	Lip endings are drawn downwards	No expression	No expression	Lips are slightly tense or stretched and drawn back	Lips are pressed together with corners straight or down, or open	Upper lip is raised Lower lip is raised and pushed up to upper lip or lowered Nose is wrinkled
Boundary portion of face	Cheeks are raised	No expression	No expression	No expression	No expression	No expression	Cheeks are raised
Fore head	No expression	No expression	No expression	Horizontal wrinkles across forehead	Forehead wrinkles drawn to the center	No expression	No expression
Mouth	No expression	No expression	No expression	Jaw drops open or stretching of the mouth	Mouth is open	No expression	No expression

FACS consists of 44 AUs, including those for head and eye positions. AUs are anatomically related to contraction of specific facial muscles, which can occur either singly or in combinations. AU combinations may be additive, in which case the combination does not change the appearance of the constituents, or not additive, in which case the appearance of the constituents changes (analogous to coarticulation effects in speech). For AUs that vary in intensity, a five-point ordinal scale is used to measure the degree of muscle contraction. Although the number of individual AUs is small, more than 7,000 combinations of AUs have been observed. FACS provides the necessary details required to describe a facial expression. In 2002 a new version of FACS was finally published, with large contributions by Joseph Hager.[14] In the new version some of the redundant AUs were removed and some were added. The system has not been renamed in the new version; it is still simply known as FACS, not as FACS2 or any other variation. The website of Paul Ekman's lab refers to it as the "new" FACS.

FACS is an analysis of the anatomical basis of facial movement. Since every facial movement is the result of muscular action, a comprehensive system could be obtained by discovering how each muscle of the face acts to change visible appearance. With that knowledge it is possible to analyze any facial movement into anatomically based minimal AUs, such as AU1 for inner brow raiser, AU2 for outer brow raiser, etc.[15] Examples of face AUs are shown in Fig. 5.2.

5.2.1.1.3 AVAILABLE DATABASES OF FACIAL EXPRESSIONS

5.2.1.1.3.1 eNTERFACE05 eNTERFACE05, hosted by Faculté Polytechnique de Mons, TCTS Lab, Belgium, includes a database of facial expressions consisting of real-time audio-visual depictions of emotions. It is a reference database for testing and evaluating video, audio, and

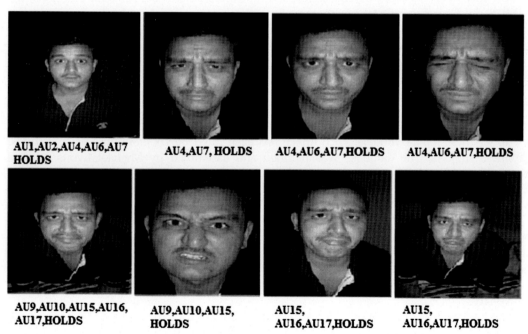

| AU1,AU2,AU4,AU6,AU7 HOLDS | AU4,AU7, HOLDS | AU4,AU6,AU7,HOLDS | AU4,AU6,AU7,HOLDS |

| AU9,AU10,AU15,AU16, AU17,HOLDS | AU9,AU10,AU15, HOLDS | AU15, AU16,AU17,HOLDS | AU15, AU16,AU17,HOLDS |

FIGURE 5.2   Some examples of AUs from FACS.

joint audio-visual emotion recognition algorithms, person identification, and audio-visual speech recognition. The videos available in eNTERFACE05 are in compressed form.[16]

5.2.1.1.3.2 COHN-KANADE AU-CODED EXPRESSION DATABASE Designed in 2001, the Cohn-Kanade AU-Coded Facial Expression Database is for research in automatic facial image analysis and synthesis, and for perceptual studies. The dataset includes subjects ranging in age from 18 to 30 years; 65 percent are female, 15 percent are African-American, and 3 percent Asian or Latino. The experiment room has a chair plus two Panasonic WV3230 cameras, each connected to a Panasonic S-VHS-AG-7500 video recorder with a synchronized time-code generator. Subjects were instructed to perform a series of 23 facial displays that include single AUs. The mean kappa for inter-observer agreement was 0.86. Image sequences from neutral to target display were digitized into 640 by 480 or 490 pixel arrays with 8-bit precision for grayscale values.[17]

5.2.1.1.3.3 MMI FACIAL EXPRESSION DATABASE The MMI Facial Expression Database aspires to provide a large volume of visual data on facial expressions. A major issue hindering new developments in the field of automatic human behavior analysis in general, and recognition in particular, is the lack of databases with displays of behavior and affect. To address this problem, the MMI Facial Expression database was conceived in 2002 as a resource for building and evaluating facial expression recognition algorithms. The database addresses a number of key omissions in other databases of facial expressions. In particular, it contains recordings of the full temporal pattern of facial expressions, from neutral, through a series of onset, apex, and offset phases, and back again to a neutral face.

Secondly, whereas other databases focused on expressions of the six basic emotions, the MMI Facial Expression Database contains both these prototypical expressions and expressions with a single FACS AU activated, for all existing AUs and many other action descriptors. Recently, recordings of naturalistic expressions have also been added.

This database is a collection of 2,900 videos and high-resolution still images of 75 subjects, and is fully annotated.[18]

5.2.1.1.3.4 JAPANESE FEMALE FACIAL EXPRESSION (JAFFE) DATABASE The database consists of 213 images of seven facial expressions (six basic expressions and one neutral) posed by 10 Japanese female models. Each image has been rated on six emotion adjectives by 60 Japanese subjects. The database was planned and assembled by Michael Lyons, Miyuki Kamachi, and Jiro Gyoba. The photos were taken at the Psychology Department in Kyushu University.[19]

5.2.1.1.3.5 RADBOUD FACES DATABASE The Radboud Faces Database is a set of pictures of 67 models (including Caucasian males and females, and Caucasian boys and girls) displaying eight emotional expressions. The database is an initiative of the Behavioral Science Institute of Radboud University Nijmegen, located in the Netherlands, and can be used freely for noncommercial scientific research by researchers who work for an officially accredited university.

The Radboud is a high-quality faces database containing pictures of eight emotional expressions. Accordingly to FACS, each model was trained to show expressions of anger, disgust, fear, happiness, sadness, surprise, contempt, and neutral. Each emotion was shown with three different gaze directions, and all pictures were taken from five camera angles simultaneously.[20]

5.2.1.2 Body Movement/Gesture

Posture in the human body is thought to be a "kind of language;[21] it has been found to be remarkably powerful in both expressing and recognizing emotion, and a strong source of information to reveal the goals, intentions, and emotions of individuals.[22]

Body language is the exposure of an emotion. Body language includes gestures, body movements (specifically leg and foot), eye behavior, posture, body position, and mannerisms.[23]

The gaze and facial expressions to convey or interpret an interaction without using words are also considered as body language, as they may provide clues to a nation of judgment.

Body language is considered to be a universal form of nonverbal communication, and helps us to understand individuals' emotions better. Information on people's emotions can be sent or received through nonverbal communication or body language. Individuals may be able to understand other individuals' emotion better by being able to recognize and interpret their body language.

Body language can express our state of mind through unconscious movements and positions. For example, if we doubt something we hear, we may raise an eyebrow; a scratch of the nose may indicate we are puzzled; shrugging the shoulders may mean lack of interest, concern or sympathy; a gentle hit to the forehead with our hand may mean we forgot something; and individuals who dislike being the center of attention may fiddle with their hands or rub them together, or rock from side to side.[24] Some examples of hand gestures used in body language are shown in Fig. 5.3.

5.2.1.2.1 FEATURES FOR BODY MOVEMENT/GESTURE

Table 5.2 gives some examples of body language expressing different emotions.

5.2.1.2.2 SOFTWARE USED FOR BODY GESTURE/MOVEMENTS

5.2.1.2.2.1 Cube26 Cube26 has a unique and sophisticated technology that is designed to deliver a fully integrated natural vision control software solution. Presence detection, natural gesture recognition, gaze tracking, face/body recognition, age/gender identification,

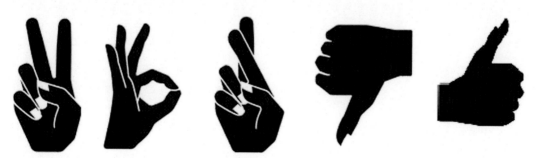

FIGURE 5.3   Different hand gestures expressing emotions.

TABLE 5.2 Feature Extraction From Body Movement/Gesture Showing Different Emotional States

Components for body gesture/ movements	Emotions						
	Happy	Sad	Neutral	Surprise	Fear	Anger	Disgust
Handedness	Hands clapping	Covering the face with both hands Hands over the head Dropping of shoulders, hands closed, move slowly two hands touching the head move slowly One hand touching the neck, moving hands together, closed	Hands on table, relaxed	Right/left hand going to the head Both hands going to the head Moving the right/left hand up Two hands touching the head Two hands touching the face, mouth right/left hand touching the face, mouth Both hands over head Right/left hand touching face Self-touch, two hands covering the cheeks Self-touch, two hands covering the mouth	Hand covering the head, body shift-backing Hand covering the neck, body shift-backing Hands covering the face Both hands over head Self-touch (disbelief), covering the face with hands	Hands on hips/ waist closed hands/clenched fists lift right/left hand up Finger point with right/left hand, shake the finger/hand crossing the arms	Backing, hands covering the head Backing, hands covering the neck Backing, right/left hand on the mouth Backing, move right/left hand up
Palm orientation	No expression	No expression	No expression	No expression	No expression	Palm-down gesture	No expression
Body movements	Body extended Arms lifted up or away from the body with hands made into fists	Contracted/closed body Dropped shoulders Body shift-forward, leaning trunk Self-touch (disbelief)/covering the body Arms around the body/shoulders Body extended			Body contracted Closed body/closed hands/clenched fist Body contracted, arms around the body Self-touch (disbelief)/covering the body parts/arms around the body/shoulders Body shift-backing	Open/ expanded body Neck and/or face are red or flushed	Hands close to the body Body shift-backing Orientation changed/moving to the right or left
Head movement	No expression	Bowed head Head bent	No expression	Head shaking, body shift-expression backing	No expression	No expression	No expression

emotion detection, and gaming interaction software make the communication between users and devices natural and seamless.[25]

5.2.2 Behavioral

Behavioral science is the systematic analysis and investigation of human and animal behavior through controlled, naturalistic observation and disciplined scientific experimentation. It attempts to draw legitimate, objective conclusions through rigorous formulations and observation. Examples of behavioral sciences include psychology, psychobiology, criminology, and cognitive science.[26]

5.2.2.1 Speech

Speech is the most natural and convenient form of communication, and the most conspicuous and basic mode of communication among humans. Speech sounds are generated by air pressure vibration produced in the lungs. The feature values of speech signals describe more than the meaning of spoken words. The goal of speech processing is to generate the sequence of words, analyze and extract the features, and recognize the speech with different modes. There are different applications in which speech signals are used: travel information or reservations, translators, virtual classes, and many more.

There are different types of speech recognition systems.

- Isolated word: obtains a single word or single utterance at one time.
- Connected words: similar to isolated word, but allows separate utterances with proper pauses.
- Continues speech: the speaker speaks almost naturally.
- Spontaneous speech: a more natural mode in which people communicate with each other.[27]

The recognition of emotion using speech is a compound and complicated effort. The vocal emotions may be induced or acted from real life. The first study of speech emotion recognition was conducted in the mid-1980s using statistical properties of certain acoustic features.[28] Emotions allow people to precise themselves beyond verbal domain. Emotion recognition from speech has gained wide attention.[29–30] Research focuses on the study of speech signal performance: how speech is modulated when a speaker's emotion changes from neutral to another emotional state.

It has been observed that speech in anger and happiness shows longer utterance duration, higher pitch, and energy value with deep length.[31] A study has also been carried out to extract features from speech to recognize emotions using various classification techniques.[32] There are distinct parameters used in this research, including mean, standard deviation, variance, and covariance; here we concentrate on pitch, intensity, and Root Means Square (RMS) energy as these give a deep sense of emotions.

5.2.2.1.1 FEATURES FOR SPEECH SIGNALS

Parameters like pitch, energy, and intensity play an important role in expressing speech emotionally. We focus on speech parameters which are also used to determine the emotions.

- Pitch. Pitch is an important parameter for speech. The pitch values contain the speaker-specific information. The pitch variation carries the intonation signal associated with rhythms of speech, speaking manner, emotions, and accent. Gender is one factor which conveys part of the characterization of the vocal tract: the average pitch for females is about 200 Hz, and for males it is about 110 Hz. In pitch variation, emotion signals in voice is one indicator, for example, speech like excitement, stress can be easily justified. Pitch variation is often correlated with loudness in speech; happiness, fear, and many other emotions are signaled by fluctuations of voice pitch.
- Intensity. The correlation of physical energy and the degree of loudness of a speech sound is intensity. The measure of amplitude via a microphone signal of a person's voice fluctuation gives the intensity of that signal. The intensity reflects watts divided by a unit area, because it is describing how much energy has radiated.
- RMS energy. RMS energy is the best signal parameter to separate emotion classes; it is used to measure the energy while speaking. The energy also affects the performance of the acoustic model in speech recognition. The voiced frame was determined by calculating the energy contained within certain bandwidths.[33]

5.2.2.1.2 FEATURES FOR SPEECH

The features extracted from speech signals corresponding to different emotions are summarized in Table 5.3.

5.2.2.2 *Text*

Detecting the emotional state of a person by analyzing a text document written by him/her appears challenging, but it is often essential due to the fact that most of the time textual expressions are directly using emotion words. Results can also be produced by interpretation of the meaning of concepts and interaction of concepts described in the text. Recognizing the emotion in the text plays a key role in human—computer interaction.[34] Sufficient work has been done regarding speech and facial emotion recognition, but text-based emotion recognition systems still need the attention of researchers.[35] In computational linguistics, the detection of human emotions in text is becoming increasingly important from an application point of view.

Since there is no standard emotion word hierarchy, the focus is on related research about emotion in the cognitive psychology domain. In 2001 W. Gerrod Parrot[36] wrote a book titled *Emotions in Social Psychology*, in which he explained the emotion system and formally

TABLE 5.3   Features Extracted From Speech for Different Emotional States

	Emotions				
	Anger	**Happiness**	**Sadness**	**Fear**	**Disgust**
Pitch	Much wider	Much wider	Slightly narrow	Much wider	Slightly narrow
Intensity	Higher	Higher	Lower	Normal	Lower
Energy	Much higher	Much higher	Much lower	Lower	Lower

classified human emotions through an emotion hierarchy in six classes at primary level: love, joy, anger, sadness, fear, and surprise. Certain other words fall in secondary and tertiary levels.

5.2.2.2.1 FEATURES EXTRACTED FROM TEXT

5.2.2.2.1.1 GRAPHICS IMAGES (GI) FEATURES

* Emotion words.
* Positive words.
* Negative words.
* Interjection words.
* Pleasure words.
* Pain words.

5.2.2.2.1.2 WORDNET-AFFECT FEATURES

* Happiness words.
* Sadness words.
* Anger words.
* Disgust words.
* Surprise words.
* Fear words.

5.2.2.2.1.3 OTHER FEATURES

* Emoticons.
* Exclamation ("!") marks.
* Question ("?") marks.[37]

5.2.3 Brain Signals and Imaging

Neurons are the cells that pass chemical and electrical signals along the pathways in the brain. They come in many shapes and sizes. Their shapes and connections help them carry out specialized functions, such as storing memories or controlling muscles. Information from one neuron flows to another neuron across a small gap called a synapse (SIN-aps). At the synapse, electrical signals are translated into chemical signals to cross the gap. Once on the other side, the signal becomes electrical again.

One sending neuron can connect to several receiving neurons, and one receiving neuron can connect to several sending neurons. As the brain is the central processing unit of the human body, its study using various techniques helped researchers to understand cognition.[38] Basically there are two ways to study the structural and functional aspects of the brain.

* **Single cell recording**. Single cell recording is significant, as it involves invasive activities. It includes brain surgery, which is stressful for the patients.
* **Brain imaging**. There are various brain imaging techniques which reveal the functions of the brain. Imaging is becoming an increasingly important tool in both research and clinical care. Many imaging methods are noninvasive and allow dynamic processes to be monitored over time. There are three main categories, often referred to as structural, functional, and molecular imaging.

5.2.3.1 Positron Emission Tomography

A brain positron emission tomography (PET) scan is an imaging test of the brain. It uses a radioactive substance called a tracer to look for disease or injury in the brain. The scan captures images of brain activity after radioactive tracers have been absorbed into the bloodstream and are "attached" to compounds like glucose (sugar). Glucose is the principal fuel of the brain. Active areas of the brain utilize glucose at a higher rate than inactive areas. When highlighted under a PET scanner, this allows brain specialists to see how the brain is working and helps them detect any abnormalities. PET scans are also used to help plan operations, such as a coronary artery bypass graft or brain surgery for epilepsy. They can also help to diagnose conditions that affect the normal workings of the brain, such as dementia.[39]

5.2.3.2 Magnetic Resonance Imaging

Magnetic resonance imaging (MRI) is a noninvasive test that helps physicians diagnose and treat medical conditions. MRI uses a powerful magnetic field, radio frequency pulses, and a computer to produce detailed pictures of organs, soft tissues, bone, and virtually all other internal body structures.[40]

5.2.3.3 Magnetoencephalography

Magnetoencephalography (MEG) is a noninvasive technique for recording brain activity. MEG has been used to study neuronal change and reorganization following stroke, head trauma, and drug administration. It is based on the detection of the magnetic fields that are generated by the currents flowing in neurons. MEG does not rely on secondary effects induced by brain activity, but directly measures the magnetic fields primarily generated by postsynaptic neuronal ionic currents.

MEG signals are reference-free and essentially unaffected by conductivity differences on the magnetic flux, providing an almost undistorted view of brain activity, and simplifying data analysis and interpretation of patterns.

MEG is a direct measure of brain function, unlike functional measures such as functional MRI, PET, and Single Photon Emission Computed Tomography (SPECT) that are secondary measures of brain function reflecting brain metabolism.[41]

5.2.3.4 Functional Magnetic Resonance Imaging

Functional magnetic resonance imaging (fMRI) is a technique for measuring brain activity. It works by detecting the changes in blood oxygenation and flow that occur in response to neural activity: when a brain area is more active it consumes more oxygen, and to meet this increased demand blood flow increases to the active area. fMRI can be used to produce activation maps showing which parts of the brain are involved in a particular mental process. It has excellent spatial and good temporal resolution.[42]

5.2.3.5 NIRS

Near Infrared Spectroscopy (NIRS) is an optical spectroscopy method that employs infrared light to characterize noninvasively acquired fluctuations in cerebral metabolism during neural activity. NIRS data consists of a series of time-dependent signals measured between individual light source and detector positions on a probe. NIRS has employed various visual, auditory, and somatosensory stimuli to identify areas of the brain associated with certain cognitive functions; other areas of investigation have included the motor system and language. The technique could also contribute to the diagnosis and treatment of depression, schizophrenia, and Alzheimer's disease.[43]

5.2.3.6 Electroencephalography

Electroencephalography (EEG), introduced in 1924 by Hans Berger, relates to electric potential in different regions. EEG is a noninvasive method, which was considered important. The EEG signals are recorded using electrical activity of the brain from the scalp. The EEG activity is small, measured in microvolts (mV). Brain cells continually send messages to each other that can be picked up as small electrical impulses on the scalp. The process of picking up and recording the impulses is known as an EEG.

EEGs can be used to help diagnose and manage a number of different medical conditions, including:

- seizures (epilepsy)
- memory impairment, such as dementia
- infections, such as encephalitis (brain inflammation)
- coma.

The different types of EEG are explained below.

5.2.3.6.1 ROUTINE EEG
- A routine EEG recording lasts for about 20–40 min.
- During the test, the subject is asked to rest quietly and from time to time to open or close the eyes. In most recordings the subject is asked to breathe deeply in and out for about 3 min.
- At the end of the procedure, with the approval of the subject, a strobe light will be placed nearby and the subject will see bright flashes of light which are repeated at different speeds.

5.2.3.6.2 SLEEP EEG
- A sleep EEG is carried out while the subject is asleep. It may be used if a routine EEG does not show any conclusive features, or to test for sleep disorders.
- While the subject is asleep his/her brain-wave patterns change significantly, and useful information related to his/her condition can be obtained. If necessary, to promote sleep, the subject may be asked to stay awake during the preceding night.

5.2.3.6.3 AMBULATORY EEG
- An ambulatory EEG is where brain activity is recorded throughout the day and night, over a period of one or more days.
- The subject is given a small portable EEG recorder that can be clipped on to his/her clothing. It records the EEG activity during the whole day and night.

TABLE 5.4   Active Regions as Features From EEG Using Different Emotional States

	Emotions						
	Happy	**Sad**	**Neutral**	**Surprise**	**Fear**	**Anger**	**Disgust**
Active regions	Prefrontal, frontal, temporal occipital	Prefrontal, frontal, temporal occipital	Occipital, frontal	Prefrontal, frontal, temporal parietal	Frontal, temporal central	Frontal, temporal central parietal occipital	Frontal, central parietal

5.2.3.6.4 VIDEO TELEMETRY

Video telemetry, also known as video EEG, is a special type of EEG that simultaneously videos the subject and records his/her brain-wave activity.

- Video telemetry is used when an EEG and continuous intensive monitoring are needed. For example, it can be used to see what a child is doing while he/she is having a seizure. This can help to diagnose the type of epilepsy that the child has, where the seizure starts, and how the electrical activity spreads through the brain.
- Video telemetry is usually carried out on an in-patient basis in a purpose-built hospital suite. It usually takes place day and night for up to five days, unless enough information about the seizure is recorded over a shorter period.[44]

5.2.3.7 Features for EEG

Table 5.4 describes active regions as features from EEG using different emotional states.

5.2.3.8 Available Online Database for EEG With Respect to Emotions

5.2.3.8.1 DATASET FOR EMOTION ANALYSIS USING EEG, PHYSIOLOGICAL, AND VIDEO SIGNALS (DEAP)

This is a multimodal dataset for the analysis of human affective states having EEG and peripheral physiological signals. A novel method for stimuli selection was used, utilizing retrieval by affective tags from the last.fm website, video highlight detection, and an online assessment tool.[45]

5.3 CONCLUSION

In this chapter we discuss emotion with respect to various modalities, which fall into the categories of physiological, behavioral, and electrical. Face, body gestures, speech, text, and various brain imaging techniques as modalities are explained. Features associated with these modalities are also described, and the available databases.

References

1. AlMejrad AS. Human emotions detection using brain wave signals: a challenging. *Eur J Sci Res*. 2010;44(4): 640−659. ISSN:1450−216X.
2. Modality. https://en.wikipedia.org/wiki/Modality_(semiotics).

3. Mehrabian A. Communication without words. *Psychol Today.* 1968;2(4):53–56.
4. Piatkowska E. *Facial Expression Recognition System.* Technical Reports. Paper 17. 2010.
5. Jiang X, Chen Y-F. Facial image processing. *SCI.* 2008;91:29–48.
6. Lee YH. Detection and recognition of facial emotion using Bezier curves. *INPRA.* June 2013;1(2):11–19.
7. Patil R, Patil CG. Automatic face emotion recognition and classification using Genetic Algorithm. *IOSR-JEEE.* September–October 2014;9(5):63–68. e-ISSN:2278-1676, ISSN:2320-3331. Ver. II.
8. Perveen N, Gupta S, Verma K. Facial expression classification using statistical, spatial features and neural network. *Int J Adv Eng Technol.* July 2012;4.
9. Ekman P, Friesen W. *Facial Action Coding System: a Technique for the Measurement of Facial Movement.* Palo Alto: Consulting Psychologists Press; 1978.
10. Ekman P, Friesen WV. *Manual for the Facial Action Coding System.* Consulting Psychologists Press; 1977.
11. FACS. http://en.m.wikipedia.org/wiki/Facial_Action_Coding_System.
12. Fasel B, Luettin J. Automatic facial expression analysis: a survey. *Pattern Recogn.* Sep 16, 2015;36(1):259–275.
13. Hussain S. *Emotion Detection from Frontal Facial Image, a thesis report, Supervisor: Abu Mohammad Hammad Ali;* 2013.
14. Vick SJ, Waller BM, Parr LA, Smith MCP, Bard KA. A cross-species comparison of facial morphology and movement in humans and chimpanzees using the Facial Action Coding System (FACS). *J Nonverbal Behav.* 2006;31(1):1–20.
15. Zaman M, Islam I. Comparative Analysis of Emotion Recognition Methods, a thesis submitted to the Department of Computer Science and Engineering of BRAC University. April 2009.
16. The eNTERFACE'05 EMOTION Database. http://www.enterface.net/enterface05/main.php?frame=emotion.
17. Cohn-Kanade AU-Coded Facial Expression Database. https://www.ri.cmu.edu/research_project_detail.html?project_id=421&menu_id=261.
18. MMI Facial Expression Database. http://mmifacedb.eu/.
19. The Japanese Female Facial Expression (JAFFE) Database. http://www.kasrl.org/jaffe.html.
20. Radboud Faces Database. http://www.socsci.ru.nl:8180/RaFD2/RaFD?p=main.
21. Mattsson. http://www.physics.leeds.ac.uk/index.php?id=263&uid=1193.
22. Kana RK, Travers BG. Neural substrates of interpreting actions and emotions from body postures. *Soc Cogn Affect Neurosci.* 2012;7:446–456. http://dx.doi.org/10.1093/scan/nsr022.
23. Mehrabian A. Significance of posture and position in the communication of attitude and status relationships. *Psychol Bull.* 1969;71:359–372.
24. Motivation and emotions. https://en.wikiversity.org/wiki/Motivation_and_emotion/Book/2011/Emotion_and_body_language.
25. Cube26. http://www.cube26.com/technology.html.
26. Behavioral Science. https://en.wikipedia.org/wiki/Behavioural_sciences.
27. Gaikwad S, Gawali B. A review on speech recognition techniques. *Int J Comput Appl.* November 2010. ISSN:0975-8887.
28. Kim EH, Hyun KH. Speech emotion recognition using eigen-FFT in clean and noisy environments. In: *16th IEEE International Conference on Robot & Human Interactive Communication, Korea.* August 2006.
29. Abhang P, Rao SA, Gawali B, Rokade P. Emotion recognition using speech and EEG signal – a review. *Int J Comput Appl.* February 2011;15(3). ISSN:0975-8887.
30. Anusuya MA, Katti SK. Speech recognition by machine: a review. *Int J Comput Sci Inf Secur.* 2009;6(3).
31. Yildirim S, Bulut M, Lee CM. *An Acoustic Study of Emotions Expressed in Speech.* Los Angeles: Integrated Media Systems Centre; 2004.
32. Ingale AB, Chaudhari DS. Speech emotion recognition using Hidden Markov Model and Support Vector Machine. *Int J Adv Eng Res Studies.* e-ISSN:2249-8974. April–June, 2012.
33. van Lieshout P. *PRAAT Short Tutorial A basic introduction;* Oct 2003.
34. Cowie R, Douglas-Cowie E, Tsapatsoulis N, Votsis G, Kollias S. Emotion recognition in human-computer interaction. *IEEE Signal Process Mag.* Jan. 2001;18(1):32–80. http://dx.doi.org/10.1109/79.911197.
35. Sebea N, Cohenb I, Geversa T, Huangc TS. *Multimodal Approaches for Emotion Recognition: a Survey.* USA; Dec 2004.
36. Parrott WG. *Emotions in Social Psychology.* Philadelphia: Psychology Press; 2001.
37. Aman S, Szpakowicz S. *Identifying Expressions of Emotion in Text.* TSD 2007, LNAI 4629. © Springer-Verlag Berlin Heidelberg; 2007:196–205.
38. Electrical signals. http://www.popularmechanics.com/science/health/a10582/study-electrical-signals-can-regrow-brain-cells-16856288/.
39. Bailey DL, Townsend DW, Valk PE, Maisey MN. *Positron Emission Tomography Basic Sciences;* 2005.

40. Hanson LG. *Introduction to Magnetic Resonance Imaging Techniques*. August, 2009.
41. Braeutigam S. *Magnetoencephalography: Fundamentals and Established and Emerging Clinical Applications in Radiology*. 2013.
42. fMRI. http://psychcentral.com/lib/what-is-functional-magnetic-resonance-imaging-fmri/.
43. Fernando L, Alonso N, Gomez-Gil J. Brain computer interfaces, a review. *Sensors (Basel)*. 2012;12(2):1211–1279. http://dx.doi.org/10.3390/s120201211. Published online January 31, 2012.
44. Types of EEG. http://www.nhs.uk/Conditions/EEG/Pages/Introduction.aspx.
45. DEAP datasets. http://www.eecs.qmul.ac.uk/mmv/datasets/deap/.

6

Multimodal Emotion Recognition

6.1 INTRODUCTION

Natural human–human interaction is multimodal and does not occur in predetermined, restricted, and controlled settings. In recognizing emotion, cognitive neuroscience research claims that information coming from various modalities is combined in our brains to yield multimodal determined percepts.[1] Similarly, in real-life situations different senses receive correlated information about the same external event. For the evaluation of emotional state, various viewpoints like distance, motion, and noise are considered,[2] thus when communicating vocally nonverbal cues such as hand gestures, facial expressions, and tone of voice also help to express feelings. Efforts are being made to enable computers to recognize these emotional inputs, and give precise and appropriate help to users in different ways that are more in line with the user's needs and preferences.

In an effort to make human–robot and human–computer interaction (HCI) more akin to human–human communication and enhance its naturalness, researchers have in the last decade approached the topic of automatic, computer-based emotion recognition. Information about the emotion felt by a user interacting with a computer can be used in many ways for human–machine interaction and computer-mediated human communications.[3] The skills to recognize, process, and display emotions are well acknowledged to be central to human intelligence, in particular influencing abilities such as communication, decision-making, memory, and perception.

Emotional sensitivity in machines is believed to be an important element in more human-like computer interaction. Due to the complex nature of human emotions, automatic emotion recognition has been a challenging task for many years. Humans express their emotions using many channels, such as speech, face, and hand gestures. In light of this, studies have concentrated on mixing multiple channels where data from the different modalities is acquired simultaneously. Data acquisition can be done in two ways. It can be offline or online. In case of offline data acquisition, inputs are already available beforehand and then it is preprocessed by excluding the parts where channels are corrupted or not suitable for evaluation. But in case of real application oriented online systems the corrupted data cannot be ignored and needed to be handled to get robustness in recognition. Fig. 6.1 shows the acquisition of data using different modalities.[4]

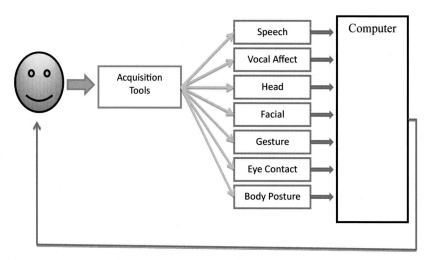

FIGURE 6.1   Diagram of a multimodal emotion recognition system.

6.1.1 The Need for Multimodal

In the last few years automatic multimodal recognition of human emotions has generated considerable interest in the research community. From a technical point of view, the challenge is in part created by the successes seen in the development of methods for automatic recognition of emotion from separate modalities. By taking into account more sources of information, the multimodal approaches allow for more reliable appraisal of human emotions. They increase the confidence of the results and decrease the level of ambiguity with respect to the emotions among the separate communication channels.[5]

Interaction between human and machine is becoming more interesting with developments in technology. Human beings communicate with each other through speech, but its verbal content does not carry all the information conveyed. Additional information includes vocalized emotions, facial expressions, hand gestures, and body language, as well as biometric indicators. From the human perspective, human–machine interaction will be more lifelike and attractive if machines are able to recognize human emotions and respond accordingly. Recognition of the user's expressed emotion can improve the reliability of communication in dialogue. Automatic emotion recognition has many important applications, including affect-sensitive automobile systems, emotionally intelligent customer services systems, and game and film industries. The field of emotion recognition has fascinated researchers from various disciplines, and current research has produced substantial advances in areas such as emotion-acquisition databases, feature extraction and selection, and classification and fusion of modalities. Earlier works primarily focused on unimodal approaches (eg, speech, facial expressions) for emotion recognition, and the modalities have largely been treated independently.[6]

These deliberations have activated investigation in the area of emotion recognition, turning it into an independent and growing field of research within the pattern recognition and HCI communities. There are two primary theories dealing with the conceptualization of emotion in psychological research. Research into the structure and description of emotion is significant, because it furnishes information about expressed emotion and is helpful in affect recognition.

6.2 MODELS AND THEORIES OF EMOTION

Emotion recognition is not multimodal but a multidomain activity. With the help of multiple cues and a knowledge of multiple subjects (psychology, computer technology, psychiatry), a robust emotion recognition technique can be developed.

In psychology various theories and models are presented and studied to mark emotions.

Many psychologists have described emotions in terms of discrete theories[7] which state that there are some universal basic emotions, though their number and type vary from one theory to another. The most popular example of this is the classification of emotions into six basic emotions: anger, disgust, fear, happiness, sadness, and surprise. This is also agreed by cross-cultural studies conducted by Ekman.[8] The advantage of the discrete approach is that in everyday life people normally describe observed emotions in terms of discrete

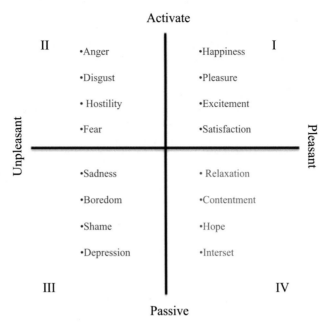

FIGURE 6.2   Distribution of emotion in a dimensional concept.

categories; the disadvantage is that it is unable to distinguish the scope of emotions which are expressed in natural communication.

There is another view known as dimensional theory, in which emotions are described in terms of dimensions. These dimensions include evaluation, activation, control, power, etc. Evaluation and activation are the two main dimensions to describe the chief facets of emotion. The evaluation dimension measures human feeling from pleasant to unpleasant, while the activation dimension runs from active to passive, and measures the likeliness of the human taking action under the emotional state. The intersection of the two dimensions is a neutral state. Russell proposed emotion distribution in two dimension which is summarized in Fig. 6.2.[7]

The first quadrant consists of happiness, pleasure, excitement, and satisfaction; the second consists of anger, disgust, hostility, and fear; the third quadrant contains sadness, boredom, shame, and depression; and the fourth consists of relaxation, contentment, hope, and interest. The advantage of dimensional representation is that it facilitates researchers in labeling the range of emotions; however, it faces difficulty in distinguishing some emotions, like surprise.

The most prominent two-dimensional models are the circumflex model, the vector model, and the positive activation—negative activation (PANA) model.

6.2.1 Circumflex Model

The circumflex model of emotion was developed by James Russell. It suggests that emotions are distributed in a two-dimensional circular space, containing arousal and valence dimensions. Arousal represents the vertical axis and valence represents the horizontal axis, while the center of the circle represents a neutral valence and a medium level of arousal. In this model, emotional states can be represented at any level of valence and arousal, or at a neutral level of one or both of these factors. Circumflex models have been used most commonly to test stimuli of emotion words, emotional facial expressions, and affective states.

6.2.2 Vector Model

The vector model of emotion appeared in 1992. This two-dimensional model consists of vectors that point in two directions, representing a "boomerang" shape. The model assumes that there is always an underlying arousal dimension, and that valence determines the direction in which a particular emotion lies. For example, a positive valence would shift the emotion up the top vector and a negative valence would shift the emotion down the bottom vector. In this model, high-arousal states are differentiated by their valence, whereas low-arousal states are more neutral and are represented near the meeting point of the vectors. Vector models have been most widely used in the testing of word and picture stimuli.

6.2.3 Positive Activation—Negative Activation Model

The PANA or "consensual" model of emotion was originally created by Watson and Tellegan in 1985. It suggests that positive affect and negative affect are two separate systems. Similar to the vector model, states of higher arousal tend to be defined by their valence, and states of lower arousal tend to be more neutral in terms of valence. In the PANA model, the vertical axis represents low to high positive affect and the horizontal axis represents low to high negative affect. The dimensions of valence and arousal lie at a 45-degree rotation over these axes.

6.2.4 Plutchik's Model

Robert Plutchik offers a three-dimensional model that is a hybrid of both basic-complex categories and dimensional theories. It arranges emotions in concentric circles where inner circles are more basic and outer circles more complex. Notably, outer circles are also formed by blending the inner-circle emotions. Plutchik's model, like Russell's, emanates from a circumflex representation, where emotional words are plotted based on similarity. In computer science, Plutchik's model is often used, in different forms or versions, for tasks such as affective HCI or sentiment analysis.

6.3 PLEASURE, AROUSAL, AND DOMINANCE EMOTIONAL STATE MODEL

The Pleasure, arousal, and dominance (PAD) emotional state model is a psychological model developed by Albert Mehrabian and James A. Russell to describe and measure emotional states. PAD uses three numerical dimensions to represent all emotions: PAD.

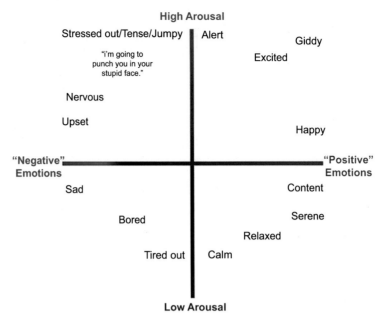

FIGURE 6.3   Arousal and valance model.

The pleasure—displeasure scale measures how pleasant an emotion may be. For instance, both anger and fear are unpleasant emotions, and score high on the displeasure scale; but joy is a pleasant emotion.

The arousal—no arousal (valence) scale measures the intensity of the emotion. For instance, while both anger and rage are unpleasant emotions, rage has a higher intensity or a higher arousal state. However, boredom, which is also an unpleasant state, has a low arousal value.

The dominance—submissiveness scale represents the controlling and dominant nature of the emotion. For instance, while both fear and anger are unpleasant emotions, anger is a dominant emotion while fear is a submissive emotion. Fig. 6.3 shows the arousal and valance model.

6.4 EARLIER EFFORTS IN MULTIMODAL EMOTION RECOGNITION SYSTEMS

In the literature various efforts are made to research emotion using multimodal entities. In chapter Emotion Recognition it is seen that modalities are categorized as physiological, behavioral, and brain signal and imaging. Combining any number of modalities is a problem to be researched. Some earlier efforts worked on various combinations of such modalities.

Facial expression is a widely researched modality in which the emotions are spotted very easily; and body movement of the subjects can also aid in revealing the emotions. A study conducted using these two modalities for recognition of emotions used full-light and point-light displays in which the body is represented by a small number of illuminated dots positioned in such a way as to highlight the motion of the main body parts. The experiment considered the emotions of happy, sad, fear, and anger, and included body posture, limb motions, body action coding system, gait velocity, and hand movements. The facial action coding system and emotional facial action coding system were examined in extracting features for facial expressions.[9]

Another study identified seven different emotions by fusing information coming from the visual and the auditory modalities. The two modalities of facial expression and voice are coupled together to identify emotions. The face definition parameters and face animation parameters were used for feature extraction for facial expressions, and for prosodic expression the voice features are the pitch, energy, formant, linear predictive coding, mel-frequency cepstral coefficient (MFCC).[10]

Yet another study recognized emotion using visual and acoustic information separately from an audiovisual database recorded from different subjects. It concluded that some emotions are better identified with audio, such as sadness and fear, and others with video, such as anger and happiness. Moreover, Chen et al. showed that these two modalities give complementary information, and argued that the performance of the system increased when both modalities were considered together. Although several automatic emotion recognition systems have explored the use of either facial expressions or speech to detect human affective states, relatively few efforts have focused on emotion recognition using both modalities. It is hoped that the multimodal approach may give not only better performance but also more robustness when one of these modalities is acquired in a noisy environment.[11]

Good research work on emotion recognition has been done on the CALLAS database, which consists of three modalities: face, speech, and gesture. The features extracted for the three modalities are as follows.

- Voice
  - Short-term features: pitch, energy, MFCC, spectrum, voice quality.
  - Long-term features: mean, median, maximum, variance, median/low/upper quartile, absolute/quartile range.
- Face
  - Short-term features: bounding box of face, positions of eyes, mouth, and nose, opening of mouth, facial expressions (happy/angry/sad/surprised).
  - Long-term features: mean, median, maximum range, position minimum/maximum, number of crossings/peaks, length.
- Gestures
  - Short-term features: acceleration and first derivative, velocity, position.
  - Long-term features: power, fluidity, volume, mean, minimum/maximum position, length.[12]

Experimental work on the audio features studied pitch, energy, duration, and MFCC features, and on visual features studied face, eyebrows, cheeks, lips, and jaws. The mouth cover distance, chin distance to mouth, nose distance to mouth, and distances of left eye to eyebrow and right eye to eyebrow are some features considered for facial expressions; and for speech, pitch, intensity, and duration were studied.[13] The identification of six basic emotions is the foal.

One study looked at the facial expression and body posture by which emotions are acknowledged. Face detection is based on action units of a face. The basic emotions (anger, disgust, fear, happiness, sadness, and surprise) are deliberated. Body postures and face expressions are combined together to get a third classifier which gives the resulting emotion.[14]

Another study analyzed face expression and speech modality. The feature mouth region was studied for facial expression. The study used a context-sensitive technique for multimodal emotion recognition based on feature-level fusion of acoustic and visual cues. The Interactive Emotional Dyadic Motion Capture (IEMOCAP) database contains detailed facial marker information used for acquiring emotions. The audiovisual database was analyzed for recognition of speech.[15]

A study of multimodal emotion recognition was performed using electroencephalography (EEG) and papillary response for the emotion categories, ie, positive, negative, and neutral. The study used the ESI Neuroscan system to acquire EEG signals, and SMI eye-tracking glasses were used for collecting eye-tracking data simultaneously. Power spectral density, differential entropy, differential asymmetry, and rational asymmetry were used for extraction of features.[16] The study detected valance from EEG signals and facial expressions in response to video. The correlation between EEG and facial expression is accomplished using continuous valence.[17] A face tracker was used for analyzing the facial expressions of the subject.

In another study, electrodermal activity, electrocardiogram, photoplethysmogram, and skin temperature as physiological signals were acquired as features and analyzed for different emotional states; 23 features were extracted from these signals and applied to four emotion classifications.[18] In other research, physiological signals like blood volume pulse, electromyography, skin conductance, skin temperature, and respiration were taken into account, studied, and analyzed to identify six basic emotions.[19]

Table 6.1 shows the efforts in this area and the multiple modalities used for the recognition of emotions.

6.5 ONLINE DATABASES OF MULTIMODAL EMOTIONS

There are several online databases available for researchers which include data on bimodal and multimodal approaches.

6.5.1 Surrey Audio-Visual Expressed Emotion Database

The Surrey Audio-Visual Expressed Emotion (SAVEE) database records the conditions for the development of an automatic emotion recognition system. Emotional behavior databases record investigations of emotions, where some are natural while others are acted or elicited. These databases have been recorded in audio, visual, and audiovisual modalities.

The SAVEE database includes phonetically balanced sentences and 60 facial markers. The database is recorded from four native English male speakers, aged from 27 to 31 years. Emotions are given categories, such as anger, disgust, fear, happiness, sadness, neutral, and surprise. The database was captured in control-flow properties of programs with procedures 3D vision laboratory. The sampling rate was 44.1 kHz for audio and 60 fps for video. The total size of the database is 480 utterances.[20]

TABLE 6.1   Efforts in Multimodal Emotion Recognition

Sr. No.	Title of research article	Used modalities
1	Development changes in emotion recognition from full-light and point-light displays of body movement[9]	Facial expression Body movement
2	Multimodel emotion recognition using EEG and eye-tracking data[16]	EEG Eye tracking
3	Bimodal emotion recognition[10]	Facial expression features, prosodic expression features
4	Exploring fusion methods for multimodal emotion recognition with missing data[4]	Facial Vocal, gestural, body approaches
5	Bimodal human emotion classification in the speaker-dependent scenario[6]	Speech Facial expression
6	Feature of multimodal emotion recognition—An extensive study[3]	Speech, facial expressions
7	Facial emotion recognition using context-based multimodal approach[14]	Facial expression Hand and body posture
8	Emotion recognition using bimodal data fusion[5]	Speech Face
9	Context-sensitive multimodal emotion recognition from speech and facial expression using bidirectional LSTM modeling[15]	Speech and facial expression
10	Continuous emotion detection using EEG signals and facial expression[17]	EEG signals Facial expression
11	Emotion classification by machine learning algorithm using physiological signals[18]	Electrodermal activity, ECG, photoplethysmogram, and skin temperature
12	Emotion recognition through physiological signals for human–machine communication[19]	Blood volume pulse, EMG, skin conductance, skin temperature, and respiration
13	Development changes in emotion recognition from full-light and point-light displays of body movement[9]	Facial expression, body movement

6.5.2 Dataset for Emotion Analysis Using EEG, Physiological, and Video Signals

This multimodal dataset for the analysis of human affective states, known as DEAP, recorded the EEG and peripheral physiological signals of 32 participants as each watched 40 one-minute excerpts of music videos. Participants rate each video in terms of the levels of arousal and valence. For 22 of the 32 participants, frontal video was also recorded.[21]

6.5.3 HUMAINE Database

A key goal of the HUMAINE project was to provide the community with examples of the diverse data types that are potentially relevant to affective computing. The database is divided into two categories: "naturalistic" and "induced."

Naturalistic data consists of audiovisual sedentary interactions from TV chat shows and religious programs, and discussions between old acquaintances. It uses 125 subjects (two sequences of 10–60 s each, one neutral, one emotional), and provides a selection of 30 sequences with ethical and copyright clearance available.

Induced data consists of audiovisual recordings of human–computer conversations elicited through a "sensitive artificial listener" interface designed to let users work through a range of emotional states. Data was collected from four users with around 20 min of speech each.[22]

6.5.4 Interactive Emotional Dyadic Motion Capture Database

The IEMOCAP database is an acted, multimodal, multispeaker database collected by the Signal Analysis and Interpretation Laboratory at University of Southern California. It contains 12 h of audiovisual data, including video, speech, motion capture of face, text transcriptors. It uses 10 actors: 5 males and 5 females. Modalities included are motion capture, face information, speech, videos, head movement, head angle information, and dialog transcriptions. Emotion categories included anger, happiness, sadness, frustration, fear, surprise, and neutral state.[23]

The verbalization of emotions is a multimodal activity. Modalities like facial expression, speech, gestures, tone, force-feedback, text, biosignals, and many more may be used for supporting robust emotion recognition systems. The approach of the study presented in this book is to investigate the correlation of EEG brain images and speech signals to examine whether these two modalities can be used as a powerful combined candidate for analyzing the emotions.

6.6 ADVANTAGES OF MULTIMODAL APPROACH

Multimodal interfaces are expected to be easier to learn and use, and are preferred by users for many applications. They hold the potential to extend computing to complex real-world applications, to be used by people. Some of the more notable advantages are as follows.

- **Robustness.** As many modalities are fused together, this leads to redundancy of information. It increases and improves communication between the user and the system, which ultimately increases the likelihood of recognition. Modalities work together to achieve a greater level of expressiveness by "refining imprecision" or modifying the meaning conveyed through another modality. The implementation of various algorithms in multimodal inputs can help to increase systems performance.
- **Naturalness.** Experimentation with different modalities results in a high degree of naturalness. Complex tasks can be eased through use of multimodal interaction, because the paradigm effectively increases the communicative bandwidth between the user and system, increasing the level of input expressivity.

- **Flexibility**. A major benefit of multimodal interfaces is flexibility, which allows the individual both to perceive and to structure the communication with respect to the context. Users can choose the modalities they want to employ.
- **Minimizing errors**. Multimodal interfaces have been proven to increase performance by reducing the number of errors (through error avoidance) and spontaneous disparities when compared to unimodal interfaces. Efficiency is not considered to be one of the major advantages of the multimodal paradigm, but users can achieve faster error correction when using multimodal interfaces.
- **Mutually adaptive**. Multimodal interfaces are ones in which both user and system co-adapt during interaction, resulting in a more predictable and synchronous whole.[10]

6.7 CHALLENGES FOR MULTIMODAL AFFECT RECOGNITION SYSTEMS

Researchers come across challenges while moving from laboratory-based experiments designed for emotion recognition to real-world systems in multimodal frameworks.

Currently existing systems have been noticed to acquire data obtained in less controlled or restricted environments (subjects taking part in the interaction may not be stationary, etc.) and can only handle a limited number of emotion categories.

The use of biopotential emotion recognition systems suffers from the drawback that they are cumbersome, may be invasive, and necessitate placing sensors physically on the human body (a sensor clip mounted on subject's earlobe, sensors mounted on the subject's head, etc.).

Moreover, EEG has been found to be very sensitive to electrical signals emanating from facial muscles during emotional expressions by the face. Therefore, in multimodal affect recognition system the simultaneous use of these modalities needs to be studied with much caution.

It is pragmatic that most researchers process each channel (visual, audio) independently, and multimodal fusion is still novel. Information from multiple channels may be ambiguous and could be misleading.

The core issue is the fact that there is a significant gap between the various groups working on research based on emotions and using multiple databases in comparison to psychology or cognitive science research groups. For justification of data a uniform and multipurpose scheme which is able to accommodate all the different modalities should be researched.

Research is still needed to answer the following questions in creating multimodal affect recognizers that can handle the so-called natural or real-world settings.

- **Number of modalities used in recognition**. Among the available external and internal modalities, will the recognition rate increase with the increase of modalities used for experimentation?
- **Choice of modality**. There are number of modalities which need proper attention, eg, tactile and visual, tactile and audio, etc., can be exploited for multimodal motion analysis. Will the chosen modality be a correct choice for consideration or not?

- How does one reach to ground truth data in posed emotions and natural data?
- Despite the advances in face analysis and gesture recognition, the real-time sensing of nonverbal behaviors is still a challenging problem.[24]

6.8 CONCLUSION

In this chapter we discuss multimodal emotion recognition. Because of certain limitations with unimodal systems, the use of multimodality must be considered to enhance reliability when adopted in real-world areas. As emotion recognition is a multidisciplinary research, psychological models are discussed in the chapter. Earlier works are acknowledged for their contributions, which help upcoming researchers to understand the basic concepts of multimodal emotion recognition. The chapter concludes by describing advantages and challenges that exist with the multimodal system, and underlines the need for doing more research in theoretical as well as experimental research to build a realistic application.

References

1. Driver J, Spence C. Multisensory perception: beyond modularity and convergence. *Curr Biol*. 2000;10(20): 731–735.
2. Gunes H, Piccardi M, Pantic M. *From the Lab to the Real World: Affect Recognition using Multiple Cues and Modalities*. May 1, 2008.
3. Paleari M, Chellali R. *Features for Multimodal Emotion Recognition: An Extensive Study*. IEEE; 2010. ISBN:978-1-4244-1674-5/08.
4. Wagner J, Lingenfelser F. Exploring fusion methods for multimodal emotion recognition with missing data. *Transactions on Affective Computing, IEEE*. 2012;2(4).
5. Datcu D, Rothkrantz LM. Emotion recognition using bimodal data fusion. In: *International Conference on Computer Systems and Technologies — CompSysTech'11*. 2011.
6. Haq S, Jan T. Bimodal human emotion classification in the speaker-dependent scenario. *Proc Pak Acad Sci*. 2015;52(1):27–38.
7. Haq S, Jackson PJB. Multimodal emotion recognition. *Machine Audition: Principles, Algorithms and Systems*. January 2010. http://dx.doi.org/10.4018/978-1-61520-919-4.ch017.
8. Ekman P. Facial Expression. In: Dalgleish T, Power M, eds. *Handbook of Cognitive and Emotion*. John Wiley & Sons Ltd.; 1999. https://www.paulekman.com/wp-content/uploads/2013/07/Facial-Expressions.pdf.
9. Ross PD, Polcon L. Development changes in emotion recognition from full-light and point-light displays of body movement. *PLoS One*. September 2012;7(9).
10. Paleari M, Chellali R. *Bimodal Emotion Recognition*. Springer; 2010.
11. Busso C, Deng Z, Yildrim S. *Analysis of Emotion Recognition using Facial Expressions, Speech and Multimodal Information*. Los Angeles: Emotion Research Group, Speech Analysis and Interpretation Lab; 2004.
12. Rehm M, Bee N, Ande E. Wave like an Egyptian accelerometer based gesture recognition for culture specific interactions. In: *Proceedings of HCI 2008 Culture, Creativity, Interaction*. 2008.
13. Haq S, Philip J, Jackson B, Edge J. *Audio-Visual Feature Selection and Reduction for Emotion Classification*. 2008.
14. Metri P, Ghorpade J. "Facial emotion recognition using context based multimodal approach", special issue on computer science and software engineering. *Int J Artif Intell Interact Multimed*. 2010;1(4).
15. Wollmer M, Metallinou A. Context-sensitive multimodal emotion recognition from speech and facial expression using bidirectional LSTM modeling. In: *Interspeech*. 2010.
16. Kheng W-L. *Multi-Model Emotion Recognition using EEG and Eye Tracking*. IEEE; 2014.
17. Soleymani M, Sadjad A-E. Continuous emotion detection using EEG signals and facial expression. In: *Multimedia and Expo (ICME)*. 2014.

18. Jang E-H, Park B-J. Emotion classification by machine learning algorithm using physiological signals. In: *Proceedings of 2012 4th International Conference on Machine Learning and Computing IPCSIT*. Vol. 25. Singapore: © (2012) IACSIT Press; 2012.

19. Maaoui C. Emotion recognition through physiological signals for human-machine communication. *Cut Edge Robot*. 2010.

20. SAVEE. http://kahlan.eps.surrey.ac.uk/savee/.

21. DEAP. http://www.eecs.qmul.ac.uk/mmv/datasets/deap.

22. Elle D-C, Cowie R. *The HUMAINE Database: Addressing the Collection and Annotation of Naturalistic and Induced Emotional Data*. 2007.

23. Ververidis D, Kotropoulos C, Pitas I. Automatic emotional speech classification. In: *Proc. 2004 IEEE Int. Conf. Acoustics, Speech and Signal Processing, Montreal*. Vol. 1. May 2004:593–596.

24. Kapoor A, Picard RW. *Multimodal Affect Recognition in Learning Environments*. 2005.

Proposed EEG/Speech-Based Emotion Recognition System: A Case Study

Introduction to EEG- and Speech-Based Emotion Recognition
http://dx.doi.org/10.1016/B978-0-12-804490-2.00007-5

127

7.1 INTRODUCTION

Chapter "Technical Aspects of Brain Rhythms and Speech Parameters" described various tools and techniques available in electroencephalography (EEG) and speech analysis. This chapter illustrates detailed implementation and experimental analysis for recognition of emotions using EEG images and speech signals.

There are various psychological tests available and used for analyzing the personality, emotions, nature, etc., of an individual. Some popular tests are the 16 Personality Factor questionnaire, the Basic Personality Inventory, the Benton Facial Recognition test, and the Emotional Intelligence Inventory (EII). The EII test[1] was used in the study for observing the emotional aspects and analyzing the emotional quotient of the subjects.

Ten subjects in the age range 22–26 were selected for our study after getting satisfactory results in the personality tests. The subjects were evaluated by emotional intelligence tests as described in chapter "Technical Aspects of Brain Rhythms and Speech Parameters". For our study, 10 out of 20 were screened out on the basis of the personality test with their consent.

The subjects were briefed and counseled about the experiments. The data was acquired in the System Communication and Machine Learning Research Lab, Department of Computer Science and Information Technology, Dr. Babasaheb Ambedkar Marathwada University, Aurangabad, India. The data for both EEG and speech were simultaneously acquired from the subjects. A corresponding database was created, from which EEG images and speech signals were selected for further processing.

Preprocessing of EEG images and speech signals was carried out, by which we were able to extract features in both types of signals. In the EEG images, a given electrode is said to be active if the acquired value of the voltage with the electrode is more than a given threshold value. In our case, this value was selected to be 30 μV. The area around the electrode which has more than or equal to the threshold value of the voltage is said to be the active region. The active electrodes were selected manually by the strength of the corresponding voltages in the regions. The Sobel edge detection technique[2] was used to get the size of the active regions in the EEG images.

For acquired speech signals, features were extracted with the help of PRAAT software.[3] The speech signals were sorted according to the emotions considered. The features considered for speech signals were pitch, intensity, and root mean square energy. A feature extraction technique was applied to get these features.

For correlating the EEG images and speech signals, Pearson's statistical correlation coefficient was applied to EEG images and speech signals. Using SPSS software, the two-tailed correlation values with their significance were calculated. The classification of three classes of mode, happy, sad, and relaxed, was performed using linear discriminate analysis (LDA). Fig. 7.1 shows the sequence of the experimental and analysis procedures for recognition of emotions using EEG and speech signals.

7.2 EXPERIMENTAL DATABASE

The creation of a database for both EEG and speech was done concurrently, as seen in Fig. 7.2. The duration of recording was 15 min for each happy and sad emotional state. During the experiment the subjects were first told to relax for about 5 min. A total of 20 EEG images were

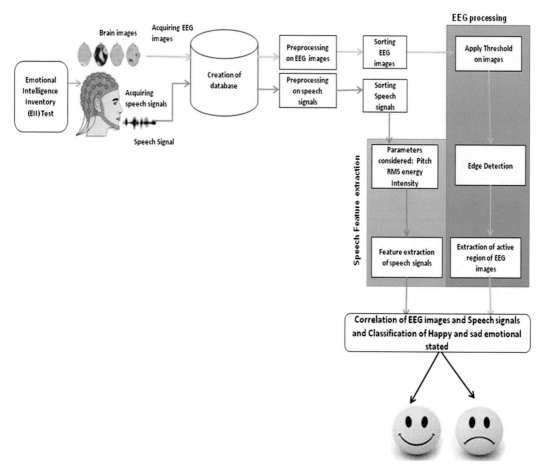

FIGURE 7.1   Procedure for emotion recognition using EEG images and speech signals.

selected for the analysis, representing average data of 45 ms. As shown in Fig. 7.2, the corresponding acquired signals were selected in a window of 45 ms. The values of pitch, energy,
and intensity from the speech signals were extracted in the selected window using PRAAT
software. For each subject, the experiments were repeated three times. Table 7.1 shows the
details of the database.

A database with the structure shown in Table 7.1 was created for the 10 subjects under
controlled conditions of relaxed, happy, and sad emotional states. As shown in the table,
three sets were created for both EEG images and speech signals. Twenty EEG images were
acquired for each subject for three sets; thus the total number of EEG images acquired was
1,800. Corresponding speech signals were used to extract values of pitch, intensity, and
related RMS energy: 20 pitch segments, 20 intensity segments, and 1 RMS energy segment
were determined for all 10 subjects for three sets, so the total number of speech signals
acquired was 2,460.

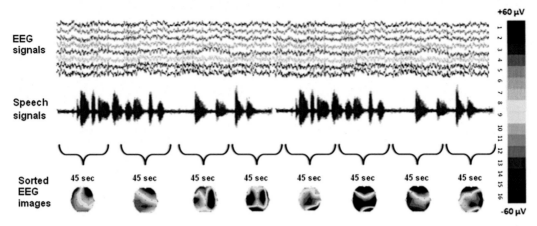

FIGURE 7.2　Creation of a database for sorting EEG images from both EEG and speech signals.

TABLE 7.1　Database for EEG Images and Corresponding Speech Signals

	No. of subjects	Emotional mental state	No. of sets acquired from each subject	No. of EEG images, pitch, intensity, and Root Means Square (RMS) energy value for mental state	Total no. of EEG images and speech signals
EEG images	10	relax	3	EEG images: 20	1,800 images
		happy	3		
		sad			
Speech signals	10	happy	3	Pitch: 20	2,460 speech signals
		sad	2	Intensity: 20 RMS energy: 1	

The machine provides brain-mapping color coding as per the international standard. The experiment used amplitude progressive, which provides 12 amplitude maps at consecutive time differences of 7.8125 ms. Fig. 7.3A shows an example of the brain images used in analysis, while the full color spectrum used in the images is shown in Fig. 7.3B.

The spectrum ranges from $+60\ \mu V$ to $-60\ \mu V$. According to the literature, $+60\ \mu V$ shows intense higher activity, and $-60\ \mu V$ shows indistinct lesser activity. There are in all 16 colors in the spectrum, but we concentrated on the first four shades, as shown in Fig. 7.4, to analyze the emotional activity in the brain.

7.3 EXPERIMENTAL ANALYSIS FOR EEG IMAGES

The EEG images were sorted out according to the significant features as determined from the regions of active electrodes, active regions, sorted EEG images, size of active region. The tables below describe the analysis of 20 images from all 10 subjects for Set 1.

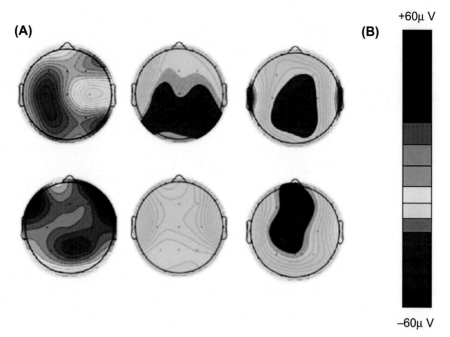

FIGURE 7.3   (A) Example EEG image, (B) Full color spectrum for EEG images.

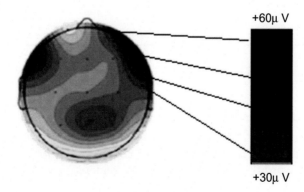

FIGURE 7.4   Selected color spectrum for EEG images.

7.3.1 Active Electrodes From EEG Images for Relaxed, Happy, and Sad Emotional States

Table 7.2 describes the percentile appearance of the active electrodes for EEG images for a relaxed emotional state for 10 subjects for set 1.

TABLE 7.2   Percentile Active Electrodes for EEG Images for Relaxed Emotional State for 10 Subjects for Set 1

Electrodes	Name of electrode	% for subject 1	% for subject 2	% for subject 3	% for subject 4	% for subject 5	% for subject 6	% for subject 7	% for subject 8	% for subject 9	% for subject 10
1.	FP1	68.42	-	5.26	57.89	36.84	-	57.89	89.47	52.63	15.78
2.	FP2	31.57	-	5.26	21.05	42.10	-	57.89	42.10	47.36	12.50
3.	O1	26.31	89.47	89.47	36.84	12.50	21.05	47.36	-	-	-
4.	O2	21.05	47.36	84.21	26.30	15.78	15.78	47.36	-	-	94.73
5.	Fz	21.05	-	-	21.05	5.26	-	12.50	15.78	-	-
6.	P4	-	26.31	-	-	-	47.36	12.50	-	-	-
7.	T6	5.26	15.78	-	-	-	31.57	12.50	-	-	-
8.	T3	31.57	-	-	15.78	12.50	-	-	-	5.26	-
9.	C3	42.10	-	-	-	12.50	52.63	-	-	-	-
10.	Cz	5.26	-	15.78	-	-	21.05	-	-	-	-
11.	C4	-	-	-	-	-	-	-	-	-	-
12.	T4	-	-	-	-	-	15.78	-	-	-	-
13.	T5	12.50	-	5.26	-	31.57	5.20	-	-	-	-
14.	P3	5.26	-	5.26	-	26.31	12.50	-	-	-	-
15.	Pz	-	-	12.50	-	-	5.26	-	-	-	-
16.	F7	47.36	-	-	-	42.10	-	-	-	52.63	-
17.	F3	47.36	-	-	42.10	57.89	-	-	-	26.31	-
18.	F4	26.31	-	-	21.05	5.26	42.10	-	21.05	42.10	-
19.	F8	12.50	-	-	15.78	12.50	12.50	-	-	-	-

Observations from Table 7.2.
1. It was observed that the FP1, FP2, O1, and O2 electrodes are more prominent.
2. Activity is larger toward the occipital and frontal regions.

Table 7.3 describes the percentile appearance of the active electrodes for EEG images for a happy emotional state for 10 subjects for set 1.

Observations from Table 7.3.
1. It is observed that the FP1, FP2, F4, F8, C4, Cz, P4, T4, T6, O1, and O2 electrodes are more active.
2. The electrodes in the right part of the brain were observed to be more dominant.

Table 7.4 describes the percentile appearance of the active electrodes for EEG images for a sad emotional state for 10 subjects for set 1.

TABLE 7.3   Percentile Active Electrodes for EEG Images for Happy Emotional State for 10 Subjects for Set 1

Electrodes	Name of electrode	% for subject 1	% for subject 2	% for subject 3	% for subject 4	% for subject 5	% for subject 6	% for subject 7	% for subject 8	% for subject 9	% for subject 10
1.	F4	**63.15**	**73.68**	63.15	**68.42**	31.57	**73.68**	73.68	**57.89**	-	42.10
2.	C4	57.89	68.42	**89.47**	68.42	31.57	5.26	73.68	42.10	-	63.15
3.	F8	47.36	63.15	63.15	57.89	5.26	57.89	42.10	57.89	-	57.89
4.	P4	47.36	57.89	47.36	-	31.57	42.10	52.63	47.36	12.50	**73.68**
5.	O2	42.10	26.31	57.89	15.78	15.78	15.78	21.05	36.84	**47.36**	-
6.	FP1	31.57	47.36	5.26	57.89	**63.15**	52.63	42.10	42.10	5.26	21.05
7.	FP2	31.57	63.15	52.63	68.42	63.15	73.68	-	26.31	5.26	-
8.	Fz	26.31	36.84	15.78	57.89	63.15	-	47.36	26.31	-	15.78
9.	T4	26.31	21.05	78.94	21.05	21.05	42.10	36.84	31.57	26.31	63.15
10.	O1	26.31	12.50	57.89	52.63	-	-	-	26.31	47.36	-
11.	F3	21.05	31.57	5.26	73.68	31.57	15.78	31.57	31.57	5.26	-
12.	T6	21.05	12.50	26.31	36.84	21.05	12.50	-	15.78	12.50	63.15
13.	T3	15.78	12.50	31.57	52.63	-	-	21.05	21.05	5.26	
14.	F7	12.50	15.78	15.78	42.10	31.57	15.78	5.26	15.78	-	-
15.	T5	12.50	-	26.31	21.05	-	-	-	12.50	31.57	21.05
16.	C3	5.26	15.78	12.50	57.89	5.26	42.10	-	5.26	-	5.26
17.	Cz	5.26	26.31	15.78	68.42	-	-	89.47	5.26	-	5.26
18.	P3	5.26	-	21.05	47.36	-	-	47.36	5.26	21.05	5.26
19.	Pz	5.26	5.26	31.57	31.57	12.50	-	-	5.26	5.26	42.10

Observations from Table 7.4.
1. It is seen that the FP1, FP2, F3, F7, Cz, P3, T3, and T5 electrodes are active.
2. The left part of the brain appeared to be more dominant.

7.3.2 Active Regions From EEG Images for Relaxed, Happy, and Sad Emotional States

The abbreviations for EEG regions are given in Table 7.5.
Table 7.6 describes the active regions of a relaxed emotional state from EEG images.

Observations from Table 7.6.
1. It is observed that the prefrontal, frontal, and occipital regions are more prominent.
2. Activity is less as compared to happy and sad emotional states.

TABLE 7.4   Percentile Active Electrodes for EEG Images for Sad Emotional State for 10 Subjects for Set 1

Electrodes	Name of electrode	% for subject 1	% for subject 2	% for subject 3	% for subject 4	% for subject 5	% for subject 6	% for subject 7	% for subject 8	% for subject 9	% for subject 10
1.	P3	**84.21**	15.78	57.89	**73.68**	26.31	-	15.78	36.84	-	**73.68**
2.	C3	84.21	42.10	63.15	73.68	12.50	63.15	47.36	-	12.50	57.89
3.	Pz	78.94	-	42.10	63.15	-	-	31.57	42.10	-	36.84
4.	Cz	63.15	21.05	5.26	47.36	-	-	**78.94**	15.78	**68.42**	36.84
5.	F3	52.63	52.63	42.10	36.84	**68.42**	21.05	15.78	15.78	26.31	-
6.	T5	57.89	31.57	68.42	15.78	26.31	5.26	-	47.36	21.05	47.36
7.	C4	47.36	21.05	15.78	15.78	-	-	-	12.50	-	26.31
8.	O1	47.36	15.78	42.10	12.50	12.50	5.26	5.26	26.31	21.05	52.63
9.	P4	36.84	5.26	21.05	12.50	-	5.26	-	36.84	-	-
10.	T3	31.57	47.36	**89.47**	5.26	12.50	31.57	-	5.26	52.6	78.94
11.	F4	26.31	12.50	12.50	5.26	5.26	-	-	-	12.50	-
12.	Fz	21.05	31.57	15.78	5.26	5.26	47.36	57.89	15.78	-	15.78
13.	T6	21.05	-	26.31	5.26	-	5.26	5.26	52.63	-	-
14.	F7	12.50	**89.47**	63.15	5.26	42.10	15.78	-	12.50	31.57	31.57
15.	O2	12.50	12.50	47.36	-	15.78	5.26	15.78	31.57	-	-
16.	FP2	5.26	47.36	15.78	-	42.10	**68.42**	5.26	31.57	5.26	-
17.	FP1	5.26	63.15	42.10	-	36.84	68.42	-	**47.36**	-	-
18.	F8	-	12.50	5.26	-	12.50	12.50	-	5.26	-	-
19.	T4	-	5.26	21.05	-	-	-	-	31.57	-	15.78

TABLE 7.5   Abbreviations for Regions

Initial abbreviation	Name of region
PR	Prefrontal
F	Frontal
C	Central
T	Temporal
P	Parietal
O	Occipital

TABLE 7.6 Percentile Active Regions for EEG Images for Relaxed Emotional State for 10 Subjects for Set 1

Sr. No.	Name of region	% for subject 1	% for subject 2	% for subject 3	% for subject 4	% for subject 5	% for subject 6	% for subject 7	% for subject 8	% for subject 9	% for subject 10
1.	F	75	-	-	75	50	40	10	25	90	-
2.	C	40	-	15	5	-	60	-	-	5	-
3.	T	15	15	-	15	15	45	15	-	-	-
4.	O	30	90	85	25	20	30	45	-	-	90
5.	P	10	25	15	-	25	55	5	-	-	-
6.	PR	75	-	5	60	35	-	50	100	100	15

Table 7.7 describes the active regions of a happy emotional state from EEG images.

Observations from Table 7.7.
1. It is seen that the prefrontal, frontal, central, and temporal regions are more prominent.
2. The activity is seen toward the right hemisphere of the brain.

Table 7.8 describes the active regions of a sad emotional state from EEG images.

Observations from Table 7.8.
1. It is seen that the prefrontal, frontal, central, temporal, parietal, and occipital regions are more prominent.
2. The activity is seen toward the left hemisphere of the brain.

TABLE 7.7 Percentile Active Regions for EEG Images for Happy Emotional State for 10 Subjects for Set 1

Sr. No.	Name of region	% for subject 1	% for subject 2	% for subject 3	% for subject 4	% for subject 5	% for subject 6	% for subject 7	% for subject 8	% for subject 9	% for subject 10
1.	F	85	100	85	100	70	85	75	85	85	80
2.	C	55	85	80	85	30	25	90	55	55	65
3.	T	50	90	70	65	30	15	80	45	50	85
4.	O	50	30	65	70	15	15	45	50	50	50
5.	P	45	95	70	50	30	20	85	45	25	85
6.	PR	45	60	60	75	65	85	45	45	-	20

TABLE 7.8   Percentile Active Regions for EEG Images for Sad Emotional State for 10 Subjects for Set 1

Sr. No.	Name of region	% for subject 1	% for subject 2	% for subject 3	% for subject 4	% for subject 5	% for subject 6	% for subject 7	% for subject 8	% for subject 9	% for subject 10
1.	F	55	100	75	60	70	75	75	30	40	30
2.	C	100	50	75	15	10	60	70	25	65	55
3.	T	90	65	80	-	30	5	5	55	80	75
4.	O	50	10	50	60	15	5	20	55	20	70
5.	P	85	60	75	15	25	5	25	55	-	95
6.	PR	5	65	40	70	40	75	20	45	50	-

7.3.3 EEG Images for Relaxed, Happy, and Sad Emotional States

Table 7.9 describes the EEG images for a relaxed emotional state.

Observations from Table 7.9.
1. A very scant area of images is seen to be active.
2. The occipital and frontal regions are active in a relaxed state.

Table 7.10 describes the EEG images for a happy emotional state.

Observations from Table 7.10.
1. It is observed that in a happy emotional state the activity is more toward the right part of the brain.
2. The prefrontal, frontal, temporal, and occipital regions are seen to be active.

Table 7.11 describes the EEG images for a sad emotional state.

Observations from Table 7.11.
1. The activity is seen more toward the left part of the brain.
2. The prefrontal, frontal, temporal, and occipital regions are seen to be active.

7.3.4 Active Region Size From EEG Images for Relaxed, Happy, and Sad Emotional States

Table 7.12 describes the active region size of a relaxed emotional state for EEG images.

Observations from Table 7.12.
1. The threshold provided for the active region size is from +30 μV to +60 μV. According to the selected spectrum, the red region of the EEG image is extracted.
2. The active region image size ranges from a minimum of 413 to a maximum of 6,354.

TABLE 7.9 EEG Images for Relaxed Emotional State for 10 Subjects for Set 1

TABLE 7.10   EEG Images for Happy Emotional State for 10 Subjects for Set 1

TABLE 7.11 EEG Images for Sad Emotional State for 10 Subjects for Set 1

TABLE 7.12   Active Region Size for EEG Images for Relaxed Emotional State for 10 Subjects for Set 1

	Subject 1	Subject 2	Subject 3	Subject 4	Subject 5	Subject 6	Subject 7	Subject 8	Subject 9	Subject 10
1	3,531	1,603	2,015	1,459	2,365	1,899	3,531	1,224	3,227	565
2	3,991	1,699	1,942	1,066	1,781	2,675	3,991	4,024	4,024	786
3	2,759	1,243	2,211	2,057	2,575	1,924	2,759	1,564	4,782	620
4	5,328	1,683	2,143	1,337	1,142	4,483	1,557	2,190	4,997	1,550
5	5,835	1,567	1,850	1,846	3,194	4,402	2,516	3,467	4,725	1,424
6	4,726	2,989	1,667	3,695	531	3,970	2,600	5,328	4,187	852
7	4,728	3,012	2,422	2,774	593	5,428	1,683	5,835	3,805	1,297
8	4,192	2,064	2,299	2,802	1,048	5,926	1,915	4,726	2,926	1,271
9	4,747	2,227	2,677	2,538	2,923	5,702	2,766	4,729	2,200	1,083
10	4,656	1,838	3,004	2,559	2,874	4,512	3,119	887	1,486	823
11	4,274	2,541	2,884	2,403	1,404	1,799	3,140	1,110	1,220	603
12	4,713	1,707	2,588	2,918	1,759	1,508	2,811	1,014	3,520	413
13	4,428	2,471	2,412	2,757	1,257	1,180	2,185	983	2,804	1,369
14	4,745	1,416	2,367	2,548	2,302	1,757	1,193	1,120	4,039	1,957
15	4,954	1,703	2,176	4,165	2,037	604	832	1,288	4,041	1,057
16	4,707	2,052	2,748	3,795	1,567	550	1,541	1,551	4,159	686
17	3,496	3,088	2,217	3,451	2,103	1,724	1,674	1,815	3,637	919
18	4,015	1,820	981	1,257	3,234	929	1,609	1,737	3,806	1,768
19	2,950	2,665	2,013	1,925	3,290	626	852	1,801	3,970	2,132
20	6,354	1,344	2,104	2,634	1,288	1,085	1,578	1,923	3,614	3,381

Table 7.13 describes the active region size of a happy emotional state for EEG images.

Observations from Table 7.13.
1. The active region size is extracted using threshold. According to the selected spectrum, the red region of the EEG image is extracted.
2. The active region image size ranges from a minimum of 2,179 to a maximum of 21,608.

Table 7.14 describes the active region size of a sad emotional state for EEG images.

Observations from Table 7.14.
1. The active region size is extracted using threshold. According to the selected spectrum, the red region of the EEG image is extracted.
2. The active region image size ranges from a minimum of 1,435 to a maximum of 20,986.

TABLE 7.13 Active Region Size for EEG Images for Happy Emotional State for 10 Subjects for Set 1

	Subject 1	Subject 2	Subject 3	Subject 4	Subject 5	Subject 6	Subject 7	Subject 8	Subject 9	Subject 10
1	6,500	6,357	7,938	13,847	4,318	5,124	4,351	13,035	4,243	12,423
2	6,161	9,281	9,603	16,059	4,469	4,395	3,573	14,089	3,473	16,091
3	9,199	6,688	9,431	16,404	4,652	5,026	13,509	11,495	3,014	8,705
4	8,657	7,134	5,636	10,719	3,277	3,969	13,091	11,265	2,250	6,298
5	6,245	7,430	7,645	21,608	5,470	4,798	10,638	11,247	3,739	8,611
6	7,009	9,275	15,588	18,724	5,172	5,538	9,636	11,402	2,683	12,254
7	7,639	6,460	11,659	15,075	4,193	5,180	13,163	10,175	3,205	14,068
8	11,018	6,094	6,058	10,718	4,614	5,913	8,390	8,561	5,390	8,591
9	10,909	5,827	4,829	9,712	4,754	6,157	13,163	9,632	3,716	5,393
10	6,432	6,126	8,935	9,853	2,998	3,764	12,329	10,245	5,168	5,986
11	5,807	5,437	8,163	15,449	2,918	3,917	8,454	10,094	6,455	5,850
12	5,326	5,476	3,680	5,799	3,799	5,632	8,729	9,608	6,616	4,404
13	5,597	6,069	10,026	4,421	5,456	5,849	9,060	5,425	6,642	4,951
14	4,882	10,781	20,117	15,742	4,935	4,072	8,419	5,582	6,079	5,676
15	4,496	9,471	15,330	14,245	4,340	3,771	8,485	4,318	6,505	5,566
16	3,629	10,872	11,142	18,357	5,468	4,841	8,390	4,160	4,662	4,883
17	3,536	12,034	8,295	13,603	4,936	5,308	8,168	4,509	4,558	4,895
18	4,053	7,034	6,628	16,023	5,012	4,650	8,159	3,463	4,598	7,406
19	3,920	8,019	5,578	5,034	4,777	3,456	9,727	2,179	6,002	3,702
20	2,668	8,925	11,276	5,191	4,690	2,885	10,436	2,608	6,070	3,624

7.4 ANALYSIS OF FEATURE EXTRACTION FROM EEG IMAGES

The feature extraction for EEG images is performed using threshold and Sobel edge detection techniques. The results are evaluated for **20 images of subject 1 for relaxed, happy, and sad emotional states for EEG images from set 1**.

Table 7.15 describes EEG active images with threshold and edge detection for a relaxed emotional state.

Observations from Table 7.15.
1. It is observed that there is much less activity in this state compared to the other two modalities, as the subjects were relaxed with eyes closed.
2. The activity is seen in prefrontal and occipital regions of the brain.

TABLE 7.14　Active Region Size for EEG Images for Sad Emotional State for 10 Subjects for Set 1

	Subject 1	Subject 2	Subject 3	Subject 4	Subject 5	Subject 6	Subject 7	Subject 8	Subject 9	Subject 10
1	13,610	4,785	6,869	4,671	4,674	1,572	3,081	6,550	15,587	7,276
2	7,887	5,180	6,469	4,167	2,556	3,631	1,667	6,075	15,484	10,130
3	10,130	4,002	6,144	4,241	2,941	3,630	1,982	6,152	14,196	9,409
4	9,409	4,020	6,069	5,417	5,141	2,048	1,823	4,761	13,460	6,402
5	6,354	3,718	6,550	5,669	3,105	3,717	2,779	4,773	13,116	5,775
6	6,875	2,199	20,986	3,428	2,565	3,706	4,270	4,788	10,723	4,933
7	10,754	7,111	11,790	4,390	1,755	2,727	4,330	5,169	11,166	6,364
8	14,064	8,612	9,970	3,962	1,843	5,289	3,644	4,502	12,239	6,936
9	15,171	6,979	9,162	3,743	5,690	5,500	3,373	4,321	13,384	6,430
10	13,932	6,434	7,557	4,091	3,720	4,507	3,237	4,455	12,459	5,659
11	11,181	4,480	5,675	2,555	2,098	5,687	2,790	3,322	12,623	9,305
12	9,294	4,725	7,082	3,491	2,344	5,715	2,522	6,067	12,079	4,595
13	9,586	3,658	5,435	4,137	1,676	4,742	3,469	8,613	13,327	5,161
14	7,139	3,597	6,769	4,201	1,969	4,709	3,740	9,413	14,172	5,272
15	7,937	3,978	5,069	4,172	2,005	4,796	2,389	8,600	4,179	5,203
16	8,208	2,360	4,837	4,045	2,284	2,026	3,486	6,154	4,520	4,816
17	11,166	13,312	7,679	4,286	2,491	1,834	4,703	4,591	4,621	5,702
18	9,641	11,458	5,217	4,538	5,185	4,977	4,376	8,065	4,167	6,524
19	6,604	9,860	12,279	4,450	4,064	4,750	2,708	9,100	5,057	8,720
20	9,914	13,974	10,938	5,078	3,553	5,102	1,435	9,170	5,884	4,690

Table 7.16 describes EEG active images with threshold and edge detection for a happy emotional state.

Observations from Table 7.16.
1. In these images the activity in a happy state is seen more toward the right hemisphere of the brain.
2. The prefrontal, frontal, temporal, and occipital regions are seen to be active. The original image with its threshold and Sobel edge detection is presented.

Table 7.17 describes EEG active images with threshold and edge detection for a sad emotional state.

TABLE 7.15 EEG Active Images With Threshold and Edge Detection for Relaxed Emotional State

Sr no.	Active happy images	Object masking (threshold)	Edge detection	Sr no.	Active happy images	Object masking (threshold)	Edge detection
1				11			
2				12			
3				13			
4				14			
5				15			
6				16			
7				17			
8				18			
9				19			
10				20			

Observations from Table 7.17.

1. In these images the activity in a sad state are seen more toward the left hemisphere of the brain.
2. The prefrontal, frontal, temporal, occipital, and parietal regions are seen to be active. The original image with its threshold and Sobel edge detection is presented.

7.5 EXPERIMENTAL ANALYSIS FOR SPEECH SIGNALS

The next series of tables describes **the analysis of 20 speech segments from all 10 subjects for set 1**.

TABLE 7.16   EEG Active Images With Threshold and Edge Detection for Happy Emotional State

Sr no.	Active happy images	Object masking (threshold)	Edge detection	Sr no.	Active happy images	Object masking (threshold)	Edge detection
1				11			
2				12			
3				13			
4				14			
5				15			
6				16			
7				17			
8				18			
9				19			
10				20			

Table 7.18 describes the parametric pitch values for a happy emotional state.

Observations from Table 7.18.

1. It is observed that the stimuli for all the subjects were similar, but the pitch value for a happy state for every individual is found to be different.
2. The parametric pitch for a happy emotional state ranges from a minimum of 138.09 to a maximum of 789.59.

Table 7.19 describes the parametric pitch values for sad emotional state.

Observations from Table 7.19.

1. It is observed that the stimuli for all the subjects were similar, but the pitch value for a sad state for every individual is found to be different.

TABLE 7.17   EEG Active Images With Threshold and Edge Detection for Sad Emotional State

Sr no.	Active happy images	Object masking (threshold)	Edge detection	Sr no.	Active happy images	Object masking (threshold)	Edge detection
1				11			
2				12			
3				13			
4				14			
5				15			
6				16			
7				17			
8				18			
9				19			
10				20			

2. The parametric pitch for a sad emotional state ranges from a minimum of 147.06 to a maximum of 571.63.

Table 7.20 describes parametric intensity values for a happy emotional state.

Observations from Table 7.20.
1. It is observed that the value for intensity differs from subject to subject.
2. The parametric intensity range for happy emotional state is from a minimum of 35.48 to a maximum of 73.69.

Table 7.21 describes parametric intensity values for a sad emotional state.

Observations from Table 7.21.
1. It is observed that the values in sad intensity are more prominent as compared to happy intensity.

TABLE 7.18   Parametric Pitch Values for Happy Emotional State for 10 Subjects for Set 1

	Subject 1	Subject 2	Subject 3	Subject 4	Subject 5	Subject 6	Subject 7	Subject 8	Subject 9	Subject 10
1	255.76	255.73	378.56	173.02	180.90	157.49	295.02	235.24	258.16	299.75
2	255.66	245.57	452.63	173.86	173.24	156.48	294.62	233.01	255.52	298.68
3	254.95	241.24	345.72	178.01	145.27	156.08	331.53	234.11	253.44	306.29
4	255.21	221.35	396.23	165.67	182.21	155.44	330.96	226.58	251.16	311.99
5	252.06	220.98	423.86	215.53	179.45	154.44	404.37	232.32	248.55	313.19
6	253.33	225.93	789.59	169.1	195.26	154.05	383.27	230.17	247.95	312.41
7	253.85	224.42	458.75	176.48	176.47	154.20	381.60	230.97	247.07	310.07
8	254.65	273.25	685.35	174.94	164.26	154.43	386.63	228.92	244.92	307.23
9	245.13	281.99	478.32	173.66	159.04	154.13	390.53	227.36	244.22	303.90
10	243.36	217.47	652.63	196.33	153.09	153.82	390.84	232.96	243.73	300.12
11	245.50	185.95	366.45	185.15	150.00	154.07	388.48	232.42	243.12	295.54
12	243.60	212.15	488.65	184.04	138.09	154.23	383.04	232.21	243.98	290.35
13	242.04	231.85	569.56	178.26	202.30	154.26	374.27	232.71	244.19	284.34
14	247.67	250.55	753.25	185.28	172.60	154.80	366.32	232.81	243.38	280.80
15	244.13	287.38	352.14	182.14	161.93	155.17	367.84	232.42	242.56	277.67
16	242.63	237.40	422.77	186.13	174.46	155.47	374.57	231.15	240.82	277.73
17	241.20	294.18	429.55	177.01	201.07	156.07	378.76	236.43	236.53	278.37
18	242.44	242.98	339.22	177.50	206.06	156.86	379.75	238.49	225.89	284.65
19	243.98	230.31	255.56	169.83	202.73	157.06	380.09	238.37	229.57	285.70
20	245.85	219.91	399.56	161.88	143.84	157.86	380.74	238.50	243.43	286.17

2. The parametric intensity range for a sad emotional state is from a minimum of 33.42 to a maximum of 88.25.

Table 7.22 describes the RMS energy values for happy and sad emotional states.

Observations from Table 7.22.
1. It is observed that the speech energy of a happy state is higher as compared to sad speech energy.
2. The parametric RMS energy range for a happy emotional state is from a minimum of 0.015 to a maximum of 0.059, whereas the range for a sad emotional state is from a minimum of 0.013 to a maximum of 0.071.

TABLE 7.19   Parametric Pitch Values for Sad Emotional State for 10 Subjects for Set 1

	Subject 1	Subject 2	Subject 3	Subject 4	Subject 5	Subject 6	Subject 7	Subject 8	Subject 9	Subject 10
1	218.75	212.90	254.81	200.15	169.34	166.36	277.01	224.94	233.92	270.55
2	213.09	200.93	255.51	204.52	169.06	166.62	278.03	224.18	233.86	268.51
3	244.62	212.43	258.88	201.97	167.08	166.55	278.56	223.98	233.47	267.52
4	227.61	266.93	251.73	200.23	165.03	167.15	279.00	223.46	236.07	267.34
5	210.30	223.40	254.75	199.80	163.73	168.64	281.37	222.85	236.52	267.64
6	218.08	210.14	259.98	194.76	163.39	169.53	284.63	223.11	229.57	267.43
7	213.05	206.64	267.29	199.14	164.03	169.34	286.06	222.41	229.58	266.70
8	219.37	229.43	250.64	203.89	164.92	170.25	287.74	223.81	232.91	266.75
9	418.79	329.96	244.24	208.49	166.03	170.86	289.09	222.84	231.70	266.83
10	313.41	317.86	243.25	212.21	167.54	171.58	290.99	222.66	238.28	266.57
11	354.02	315.59	244.83	211.92	168.89	171.92	294.31	223.26	239.00	266.52
12	264.75	296.27	252.01	213.57	169.96	172.02	298.77	224.72	238.02	265.55
13	182.72	280.39	250.36	211.43	170.80	171.50	303.99	225.05	235.72	264.15
14	219.22	357.01	248.42	199.32	172.53	170.28	309.55	224.93	234.40	262.85
15	223.31	250.47	247.93	197.01	171.74	170.57	314.37	228.42	237.05	262.64
16	219.02	324.55	252.94	195.57	167.19	171.63	317.62	228.69	238.46	263.91
17	210.30	571.63	262.10	186.30	164.85	171.66	318.96	226.86	238.81	266.05
18	176.49	382.69	253.43	187.68	153.75	171.96	317.03	223.44	241.04	268.14
19	203.85	242.47	258.93	186.44	150.36	172.05	304.05	224.41	237.72	269.16
20	246.39	296.67	262.98	185.55	147.06	171.89	290.97	225.19	236.46	269.64

7.6 CORRELATION OF EEG IMAGES AND SPEECH SIGNALS

The statistical tool available with SPSS is used for evaluation of correlation between EEG images and speech signals. The next series of tables describes the correlation between EEG images, pitch, and intensity signals for happy and sad emotional states for **set 1, set 2, and set 3.** The (*) correlation is significant at the 0.05 level (two-tailed), and (**) correlation is significant at the 0.01 level (two-tailed).

Table 7.23 describes the correlation of EEG images with happy pitch and sad pitch for set 1.

TABLE 7.20   Parametric Intensity Values for Happy Emotional State for 10 Subjects for Set 1

	Subject 1	Subject 2	Subject 3	Subject 4	Subject 5	Subject 6	Subject 7	Subject 8	Subject 9	Subject 10
1	58.45	61.50	66.45	63.11	70.29	54.14	66.87	63.39	35.48	39.27
2	58.18	60.58	66.31	63.97	70.19	50.40	67.93	63.05	36.57	39.75
3	58.14	61.29	66.98	64.22	69.38	48.91	68.75	62.48	37.81	39.41
4	58.25	60.79	69.21	64.48	67.10	48.44	69.27	61.93	38.09	38.70
5	58.28	60.68	65.56	64.30	62.92	47.59	69.61	62.04	37.75	39.06
6	58.37	60.13	64.11	63.83	58.06	46.09	69.79	62.47	38.77	39.24
7	58.86	61.16	63.58	63.52	54.77	44.61	69.78	62.81	40.69	38.18
8	59.53	60.81	60.92	64.77	51.13	43.08	69.60	62.73	41.91	37.79
9	60.12	60.99	62.88	64.23	46.72	42.39	69.38	62.71	42.52	38.64
10	60.75	61.12	54.10	64.64	44.73	45.79	69.18	62.78	43.01	38.8
11	60.94	61.03	52.24	64.81	44.87	50.26	69.00	62.88	43.19	38.38
12	60.59	60.67	47.74	64.84	49.80	53.92	68.45	63.54	43.55	38.05
13	59.92	60.74	46.56	64.91	59.24	62.18	67.54	63.97	44.23	37.55
14	58.98	61.90	46.17	63.63	66.45	68.61	67.04	63.72	44.86	37.18
15	57.91	62.51	45.30	64.09	70.78	72.03	66.85	63.05	45.19	36.84
16	56.56	62.45	50.16	63.81	72.85	73.42	67.01	62.80	45.64	36.80
17	55.32	61.71	65.93	63.96	73.37	73.69	67.88	63.39	46.10	37.50
18	54.92	60.77	66.52	64.35	72.94	73.51	69.13	64.04	46.17	37.63
19	55.30	61.03	66.06	64.33	72.04	73.19	70.06	64.27	46.13	38.26
20	56.04	60.94	59.72	64.08	70.64	72.36	70.45	64.12	46.07	40.09

Observations from Table 7.23.
1. It is observed that when the value of correlation increases the significance decreases.
2. The strength of relationship falls under a **strong** correlation.[4] It is also observed that the happy pitch is more prominent than the sad pitch.

Table 7.24 describes the correlation of EEG images with happy intensity and sad intensity for set 1.

Observations from Table 7.24.
1. It is observed that when the value of correlation increases the significance decreases.
2. It is also observed that the sad intensity is more prominent than the happy intensity.

Table 7.25 describes the correlation of EEG images with happy pitch and sad pitch for set 2.

TABLE 7.21   Parametric Intensity Values for Sad Emotional State for 10 Subjects for Set 1

	Subject 1	Subject 2	Subject 3	Subject 4	Subject 5	Subject 6	Subject 7	Subject 8	Subject 9	Subject 10
1	66.54	83.55	61.50	64.45	66.98	60.13	58.67	59.45	40.32	44.58
2	68.10	87.74	61.08	63.47	65.77	60.01	59.40	59.32	38.76	45.10
3	66.23	65.56	60.42	62.60	64.04	59.83	59.79	59.36	40.15	44.03
4	71.57	84.37	61.04	62.53	64.62	60.53	59.70	59.41	39.86	42.29
5	67.44	83.68	61.97	62.98	65.51	61.31	59.32	59.27	39.93	43.19
6	73.83	86.01	62.27	63.56	64.89	62.24	58.88	58.84	38.76	44.67
7	70.43	85.86	62.07	64.66	62.53	63.16	58.56	58.17	36.54	43.08
8	73.23	85.59	62.13	65.86	58.86	63.83	58.57	57.47	36.11	42.84
9	87.84	81.74	62.45	66.28	54.87	64.12	58.33	57.25	36.81	45.70
10	87.42	83.59	62.27	66.41	51.29	63.80	57.81	57.66	38.97	47.13
11	88.25	82.35	61.87	66.79	48.15	63.17	57.86	58.12	39.96	46.88
12	56.63	76.64	61.42	67.01	45.59	62.57	58.30	58.42	39.82	46.22
13	84.08	77.04	60.98	67.24	44.52	61.71	58.53	58.92	38.38	45.02
14	71.57	72.69	60.62	67.34	44.95	60.60	58.55	59.75	37.10	43.90
15	67.44	76.75	60.61	67.09	48.72	60.05	58.35	60.25	35.92	43.02
16	73.83	87.33	60.97	66.92	58.33	60.11	58.20	60.29	34.55	44.82
17	70.43	84.07	61.13	66.87	64.90	59.98	58.01	59.89	33.55	45.51
18	76.95	85.13	61.45	66.88	67.86	59.81	57.90	59.73	33.42	45.78
19	73.47	37.11	61.77	66.35	68.66	60.27	58.24	59.85	34.32	46.67
20	68.30	35.24	61.73	65.46	68.82	61.14	58.45	59.75	34.49	48.10

Observations from Table 7.25.
1. It is observed that the sad pitch is more prominent than the happy pitch.
2. As compared to set 1, the values are seen to be improving in set 2.

Table 7.26 describes the correlation of EEG images with happy intensity and sad intensity for set 2.

Observations from Table 7.26.
1. It is observed that sad intensity is more prominent than happy intensity.
2. The strength of relationship falls under a **strong** correlation.

TABLE 7.22   RMS Energy Values for Happy and Sad Emotional States for 10 Subjects for Set 1

Speech values	RMS energy for happy mode	RMS energy for sad mode
Subject 1	0.026	0.018
Subject 2	0.024	0.021
Subject 3	0.058	0.046
Subject 4	0.053	0.071
Subject 5	0.059	0.049
Subject 6	0.046	0.053
Subject 7	0.040	0.032
Subject 8	0.046	0.031
Subject 9	0.015	0.013
Subject 10	0.025	0.023

TABLE 7.23   Correlation of EEG Images With Happy Pitch and Sad Pitch for 10 Subjects for Set 1

Subject	Pitch for happy mode		Pitch for sad mode	
	Correlation	Significance	Correlation	Significance
Subject 1	0.598(**)	0.005	0.566(**)	0.009
Subject 2	0.400	0.081	0.495(*)	0.027
Subject 3	0.451(*)	0.046	0.458(*)	0.042
Subject 4	0.436	0.055	0.456(*)	0.044
Subject 5	0.499(*)	0.025	0.415	0.069
Subject 6	0.431	0.058	0.536(*)	0.015
Subject 7	0.443	0.050	0.438	0.053
Subject 8	0.518(*)	0.019	0.421	0.065
Subject 9	0.477(*)	0.034	0.508(*)	0.022
Subject 10	0.574(**)	0.008	0.452(*)	0.045

TABLE 7.24 Correlation of EEG Images With Intensity Parameters Corresponding to Happy and Sad Modes for 10 Subjects for Set 1

Subject	Intensity for happy mode		Intensity for sad mode	
	Correlation	Significance	Correlation	Significance
Subject 1	0.555(*)	0.011	0.417	0.067
Subject 2	0.495(*)	0.027	0.445(*)	0.049
Subject 3	0.410	0.073	0.573(**)	0.008
Subject 4	0.457(*)	0.043	0.449(*)	0.047
Subject 5	0.492(*)	0.028	0.450(*)	0.046
Subject 6	0.420	0.065	0.468(*)	0.037
Subject 7	0.553(*)	0.011	0.490(*)	0.028
Subject 8	0.676(**)	0.001	0.620(**)	0.004
Subject 9	0.694(**)	0.001	0.846(**)	0.000
Subject 10	0.423	0.063	0.498(*)	0.025

TABLE 7.25 Correlation of EEG Images With Happy and Sad Pitches for 10 Subjects for Set 2

Subject	Pitch for happy mode		Pitch for sad mode	
	Correlation	Significance	Correlation	Significance
Subject 1	0.509(*)	0.022	0.490(*)	0.028
Subject 2	0.474(*)	0.035	0.625(**)	0.003
Subject 3	0.694(**)	0.001	0.618(**)	0.004
Subject 4	0.415	0.069	0.408	0.074
Subject 5	0.481(*)	0.032	0.411	0.072
Subject 6	0.407	0.075	0.560(*)	0.010
Subject 7	0.615(**)	0.004	0.725(**)	0.000
Subject 8	0.465(*)	0.039	0.552(*)	0.012
Subject 9	0.472(*)	0.036	0.563(**)	0.010
Subject 10	0.553(*)	0.011	0.466(*)	0.038

TABLE 7.26   Correlation of EEG Images With Intensity Corresponding to Happy and Sad Modes for 10 Subjects for Set 2

Subject	Happy intensity		Sad intensity	
	Correlation	Significance	Correlation	Significance
Subject 1	0.418	0.067	0.527(*)	0.017
Subject 2	0.468(*)	0.037	0.526(*)	0.017
Subject 3	0.620(**)	0.004	0.449(*)	0.047
Subject 4	0.477(*)	0.034	0.465(*)	0.039
Subject 5	0.481(*)	0.032	0.628(**)	0.003
Subject 6	0.453(*)	0.045	0.567(**)	0.009
Subject 7	0.859(**)	0.000	0.805(**)	0.000
Subject 8	0.444(*)	0.050	0.476(*)	0.034
Subject 9	0.506(*)	0.023	0.441	0.052
Subject 10	0.511(*)	0.021	0.513(*)	0.021

TABLE 7.27   Correlation of EEG Images With Happy and Sad Pitches for 10 Subjects for Set 3

Subject	Happy pitch		Sad pitch	
	Correlation	Significance	Correlation	Significance
Subject 1	0.401	0.080	0.479(*)	0.033
Subject 2	0.502(*)	0.024	0.400	0.080
Subject 3	0.525(*)	0.018	0.502(*)	0.024
Subject 4	0.427	0.061	0.421	0.068
Subject 5	0.477(*)	0.033	0.460(*)	0.041
Subject 6	0.410	0.072	0.450	0.046
Subject 7	0.645(**)	0.002	0.534(*)	0.015
Subject 8	0.812(**)	0.000	0.602(**)	0.005
Subject 9	0.488(*)	0.029	0.681(**)	0.001
Subject 10	0.438	0.072	0.506(*)	0.023

Table 7.27 describes the correlation of EEG images with happy and sad pitches for set 3.

Observations from Table 7.27.
1. It is observed that sad pitch is more prominent than happy pitch.
2. The strength of relationship falls under a **strong** correlation.

Table 7.28 describes the correlation of EEG images with happy and sad intensities for set 3.

Observations from Table 7.28.
1. It is observed that sad intensity is more prominent than happy intensity.
2. The strength of relationship falls under a **strong** correlation.

7.7 CLASSIFICATION USING LINEAR DISCRIMINATE ANALYSIS

As described in chapter "Technical Aspects of Brain Rhythms and Speech Parameters", the main objective of using LDA is to perform dimensionality reduction while preserving as much of the class discriminatory information as possible.

We applied the LDA classification technique to both EEG images and speech signals. All three sets are described here for both modalities. The classification accuracy is computed as $(x/n) \times 100$, where x is the number of points in the cluster and n is the total number of subjects (here 10).

Fig. 7.5 describes LDA implementation for EEG images for relaxed, happy, and sad emotional states for 10 subjects for **set 1**.

TABLE 7.28 Correlation of EEG Images With Happy and Sad Intensities for 10 Subjects for Set 3

Subject	Intensity for happy mode		Intensity for sad mode	
	Correlation	Significance	Correlation	Significance
Subject 1	0.419	0.066	0.547(*)	0.013
Subject 2	0.519(*)	0.019	0.486(*)	0.030
Subject 3	0.502(*)	0.024	0.440	0.052
Subject 4	0.493(*)	0.065	0.469	0.039
Subject 5	0.428	0.060	0.490(*)	0.028
Subject 6	0.478	0.036	0.429	0.072
Subject 7	0.424	0.062	0.509(*)	0.022
Subject 8	0.629(**)	0.003	0.714(**)	0.000
Subject 9	0.474(*)	0.035	0.578(**)	0.008
Subject 10	0.458	0.056	0.424	0.063

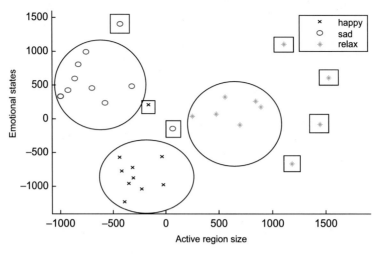

FIGURE 7.5   LDA implementation for EEG images for relaxed, happy, and sad emotional states for 10 subjects for set 1.

Observations from Fig. 7.5.
1. The relaxed, happy, and sad emotional states are resulted and seen in Fig. 7.5. The relaxed, happy, and sad emotional states are on the X axis, while the active region size is placed on the Y axis.
2. The accuracy rate for set 1 is shown in Table 7.29. It is observed that the accuracy for relaxed is 60 percent, happy is 90 percent, sad is 80 percent, and the overall accuracy is 76 percent.

Fig. 7.6 shows LDA implementation for EEG images for relaxed, happy, and sad emotional states for 10 subjects for **set 2**.

Observations from Fig. 7.6.
1. The relaxed, happy, and sad emotional states are resulted and seen in Fig. 7.6. The relaxed, happy, and sad emotional states are on the X axis, and the active region size is placed on the Y axis.
2. The accuracy rate for set 2 is shown in Table 7.30. The accuracy for relaxed is 70 percent, happy is 90 percent, sad is 90 percent, and the overall accuracy is 83 percent.

TABLE 7.29   Accuracy for Emotional States for 10 Subjects for Set 1

Emotional state	n	x	% accuracy	% overall accuracy
Relaxed	10	6	60	76
Happy	10	9	90	
Sad	10	9	80	

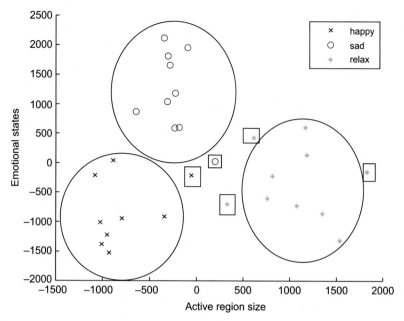

FIGURE 7.6   LDA implementation for EEG images for relaxed, happy, and sad emotional states for 10 subjects for set 2.

TABLE 7.30   Accuracy for Emotional States for 10 Subjects for Set 2

Emotional state	n	x	% accuracy	% overall accuracy
Relaxed	10	7	70	83
Happy	10	9	90	
Sad	10	9	90	

Fig. 7.7 shows LDA implementation for EEG images for relaxed, happy, and sad emotional states for 10 subjects for **set 3**.

Observations from Fig. 7.7.

1. The relaxed, happy, and sad emotional states are on the X axis, whereas the active region size is placed on the Y axis.
2. The accuracy rate for set 3 is shown in Table 7.31. The accuracy for relaxed is 90 percent, happy is 90 percent, sad is 90 percent, and the overall accuracy is 90 percent.

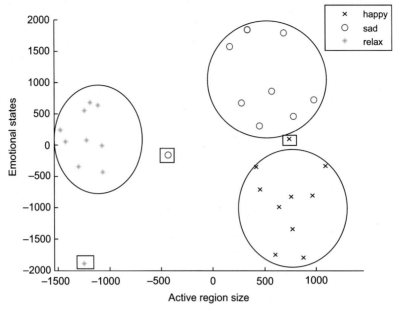

FIGURE 7.7   LDA implementation for EEG images for relaxed, happy, and sad emotional states for 10 subjects for set 3.

TABLE 7.31   Accuracy for Emotional States for 10 Subjects for Set 3

Emotional state	n	x	% accuracy	% overall accuracy
Relaxed	10	9	90	90
Happy	10	9	90	
Sad	10	9	90	

Fig. 7.8 shows LDA implementation for pitch values for happy and sad emotional states for 20 speech segments for 10 subjects of **set 1**.

Observations from Fig. 7.8.

1. It is observed that the clusters formed for happy and sad speech for the pitch parameter are distinct from each other. Happy and sad emotional states are on the X axis, with active pitch values placed on the Y axis.
2. The accuracy rate for set 1 is seen in Table 7.32. The accuracy for happy is 100 percent, sad is 100 percent, and overall accuracy is 100 percent.

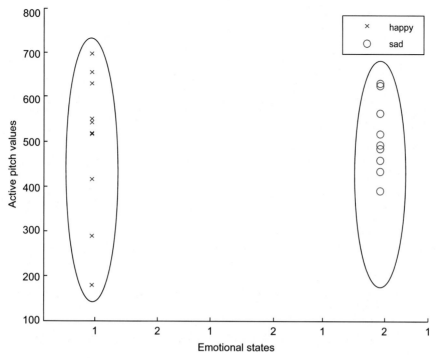

FIGURE 7.8   LDA implementation for pitch for 20 speech segments for 10 subjects of set 1.

TABLE 7.32   Accuracy for Two Emotional States for 20 Speech
Segments for 10 Subjects for Set 1

Emotional state	n	x	% accuracy	% overall accuracy
Happy	10	10	100	100
Sad	10	10	100	

Fig. 7.9 shows LDA implementation for intensity values for happy and sad emotional states for 20 speech segments for 10 subjects for **set 1**.

Observations from Fig. 7.9.

1. It is observed that the clusters formed for happy and sad speech for the intensity parameter are distinct from each other. Happy and sad emotional states are on the X axis, with active intensity values placed on the Y axis.
2. The accuracy rate for set 1 is seen in Table 7.33. The accuracy for happy is 100 percent, sad is 100 percent, and the overall accuracy is 100 percent.

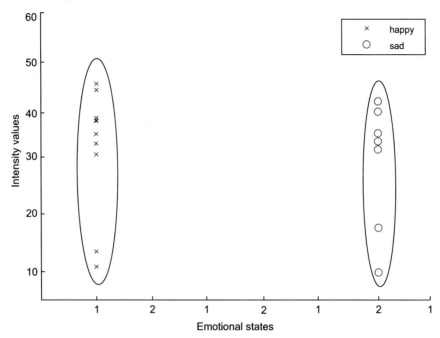

FIGURE 7.9   LDA implementation for intensity for 20 speech segments for 10 subjects of set 1.

TABLE 7.33   Accuracy for Two Emotional States for 20 Speech
Segments for 10 Subjects for Set 1

Emotional state	n	x	% accuracy	% overall accuracy
Happy	10	10	100	100
Sad	10	10	100	

Fig. 7.10 shows LDA implementation for pitch values for happy and sad emotional states for 20 speech segments for 10 subjects of **set 2**.

Observations from Fig. 7.10.

1. It is observed that the clusters formed for happy and sad speech for the pitch parameter are distinct from each other. Happy and sad emotional states are on the X axis, whereas active pitch values are placed on the Y axis.
2. The accuracy rate for set 2 is seen in Table 7.34. The accuracy for happy is 100 percent, sad is 90 percent, and the overall accuracy is 95 percent.

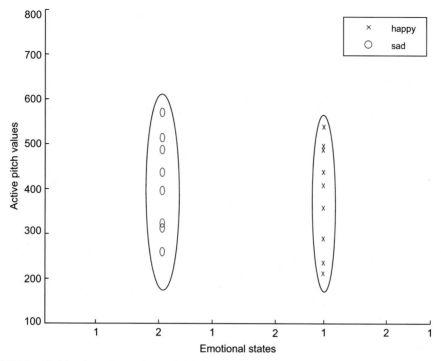

FIGURE 7.10   LDA implementation for pitch for 20 speech segments for 10 subjects of set 2.

TABLE 7.34   Accuracy for Two Emotional States for 20 Speech Segments for 10 Subjects of Set 2

Emotional state	n	x	% accuracy	% overall accuracy
Happy	10	10	100	95
Sad	10	10	90	

Fig. 7.11 shows LDA implementation for intensity values for happy and sad emotional states for 20 speech segments for 10 subjects of **set 2**.

Observations from Fig. 7.11.

1. It is observed that the clusters formed for happy and sad speech for the intensity parameter are distinct from each other. Happy and sad emotional states are on the X axis, whereas active intensity values are placed on the Y axis.
2. The accuracy rate for set 2 is seen in Table 7.35. The accuracy for happy is 90 percent, sad is 90 percent, and the overall accuracy is 90 percent.

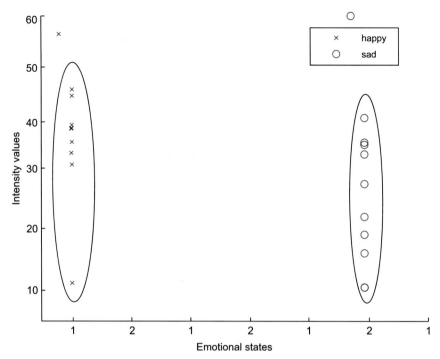

FIGURE 7.11   LDA implementation for intensity for 20 speech segments for 10 subjects of set 2.

TABLE 7.35   Accuracy for Two Emotional States for 20 Speech Segments for 10 Subjects for Set 2

Emotional state	n	x	% accuracy	% overall accuracy
Happy	10	10	90	90
Sad	10	10	90	

Fig. 7.12 shows LDA implementation for pitch values for happy and sad emotional states for 20 speech segments for 10 subjects of **set 3**.

Observations from Fig. 7.12.
1. It is observed that the clusters formed for happy and sad speech for the pitch parameter are distinct from each other. Happy and sad emotional states are on the X axis, and active pitch values are placed on the Y axis.
2. The accuracy rate for set 3 is seen in Table 7.36. The accuracy for happy is 90 percent, sad is 90 percent, and the overall accuracy is 90 percent.

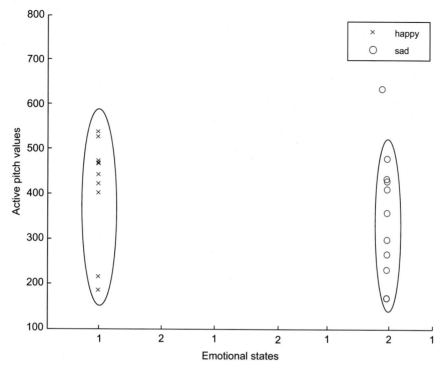

FIGURE 7.12   LDA implementation for pitch for 20 speech segments for 10 subjects of set 3.

TABLE 7.36   Accuracy for Two Emotional States for 20 Speech Segments for 10 Subjects of Set 3

Emotional state	n	x	% accuracy	% overall accuracy
Happy	10	10	100	95
Sad	10	10	90	

Fig. 7.13 shows LDA implementation for intensity values for happy and sad emotional states for 20 speech segments for 10 subjects of **set 3**.

Observations from Fig. 7.13.

1. It is observed that the clusters formed for happy and sad speech for the intensity parameter are distinct from each other. Happy and sad emotional states are on the X axis, with active intensity values placed on the Y axis.
2. The accuracy rate for set 3 is seen in Table 7.37. The accuracy for happy is 90 percent, sad is 90 percent, and the overall accuracy is 90 percent.

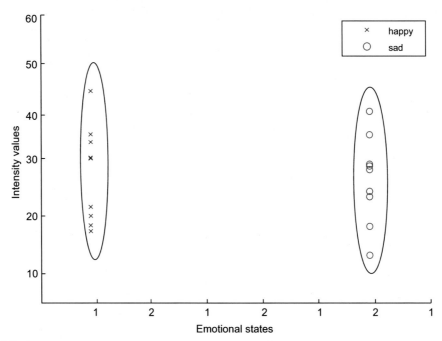

FIGURE 7.13   LDA implementation for intensity for 20 speech segments for 10 subjects of set 3.

TABLE 7.37   Accuracy for Two Emotional States for 20 Speech
Segments for 10 Subjects for Set 3

Emotional state	*n*	*x*	% accuracy	% overall accuracy
Happy	10	10	100	95
Sad	10	10	90	

7.8 CONCLUSION

Emotions are seen and observed as distinct from person to person in this chapter. Using different tools and techniques, we implemented the EII test to select subjects on the basis of emotion. Acquiring EEG images and speech signals simultaneously, we created our own database. Analysis was performed on the data collected, which was sorted according to the emotions selected for experimentation: relaxed, happy, and sad.

The features selected for EEG images were active region, active electrodes, and active region size; the features selected for speech signals were pitch, intensity, and RMS energy, which are more beneficial parameters for extracting proper emotions.

For bimodal fusion of EEG images and speech signals we used a statistical technique of Pearson's correlation coefficient and SPSS software for correlating the two modalities.

The strength of correlation for both EEG images and speech signals was found to be between moderate and strong. The correlation coefficient significance accuracy is about 95 percent for each emotional state.

By applying LDA to both EEG images and speech signals, the accuracy of the overall evaluated results is as follows.

1. Overall result from EEG images for set 1 is 76 percent.
2. Overall result from EEG images for set 2 is 83 percent.
3. Overall result from EEG images for set 3 is 90 percent.
4. Overall result for pitch and intensity for set 1 is 100 percent.
5. Overall result for pitch is 95 percent and for intensity 90 percent for set 2.
6. Overall result for pitch is 90 percent and for intensity 90 percent for set 3.

It is observed from the results that these two modalities are suitable for developing a robust emotion recognition system.

References

1. Mangal SK, Mangal S. *Emotion intelligence inventory test.* National Psychological Corporation, Estb. 1971; 2012.
2. Gonzalez RC, Woods RE, Eddins SL. *Digital image processing using MATLAB.* Pearson Education, Inc.; 2004.
3. Lieshout PV. *PRAAT Short Tutorial- A basic introduction.* V. 4.2.1. October 7, 2003.
4. Statistics in Psychology MPC-006. *Correlation and Regression.* Book no 2. Indira Gandhi National Open University, School of Social Sciences; January 2012.

8

Brain–Computer Interface Systems and Their Applications

8.1 INTRODUCTION

Brain–computer interface (BCI) systems are fast-growing emergent technologies in which researchers aim to build direct communication between the human brain and a computer. It is a collaboration in which a brain accepts and controls a mechanical device, giving a direct connection between the computer(s) and the human brain. BCI has many applications, especially for disabled persons. It reads the waves produced by the brain and translates these signals into actions and commands that can control the computer(s).[1]

BCI is a rapid-paced technology. It started in 1964, when Dr. Grey Walter successfully formed a BCI wherein he connected electrodes directly to the motor areas of a patient's brain. The experiments conducted was successful in advancing the slide through the relevant brain activity and was one of the first BCI applications. The findings were not published, but Dr. Walter presented a talk at the Ostler Society in London.[2]

The BCI can lead to many applications, most of which are related to helping disabled persons to live as normal people. Artificial intelligence and computational intelligence are two major subjects involved in BCI. Signal processing algorithms and increased computing power have reduced the need for bulky equipment. BCIs have been explored in applications as diverse as security, lie detection, alertness monitoring, gaming, education, art, and human augmentation in which technology enhances the human capability through implant and other technologies.

BCI exploits the fact that certain aspects of brain activity are linked to specific mental states and processes, called "signatures" or "features." A BCI is a combination of techniques for recording brain activity, extracting and processing signatures, and translating aspects of the signature into computer commands, which are fed back to the user. There are BCIs that partially restore movement and/or communicative capabilities in paralyzed patients,[3] as well as BCIs that explore new ways of playing computer games.[4]

Initial development of BCIs aimed to build assistive devices for physically challenged or individuals suffering from extreme loss of voluntary muscle movement (locked-in users). The technology is no longer limited only to medical applications, and has widened to include nonmedical applications.

8.2 WORKING OF BCI SYSTEMS

The operation of a BCI generally involves several steps, as seen in Fig. 8.1.

1. Acquisition to capture the signal from the brain.
2. Preprocessing to prepare the raw data obtained for further steps.
3. Signature/feature extraction.
4. Feature classification.
5. Translation of the classified signature/feature into computer commands.
6. Application interface for the actual application design.

The techniques used for these steps vary according to the application that is to be developed.

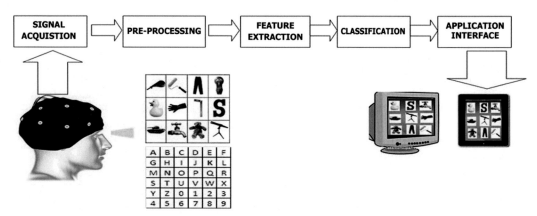

FIGURE 8.1   An example of a brain–computer interface cycle.

8.3 TYPES OF BCI

The brain can be interfaced in three major ways, as shown in Fig. 8.2.

There are several types of BCI, but the basic function of all types is to intercept the electrical signals that communicate between nerve cells in the brain and turn them into a signal that is sensed by external devices.

8.3.1 Invasive BCI

Invasive BCIs are neuroprosthetics whose electrode array heads are buried within the brain itself on a permanent basis. They have better signal-to-noise ratio and more accuracy than other BCI-based systems, but they require complex surgery to implant and usually involve a permanent hole in the skull. Fig. 8.3 shows an example of invasive BCI.

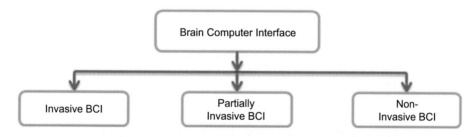

FIGURE 8.2   Types of BCI.

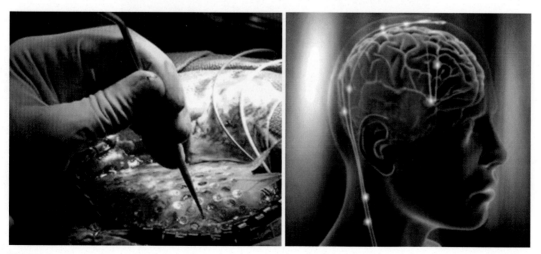

FIGURE 8.3   Example of invasive BCI.

Advantages
- Invasive BCIs generally use electrodes (sensors) that are implanted directly into the gray matter of the brain during neurosurgery.
- The electrodes lie in the gray matter of the brain.
- Invasive BCI produces the highest-quality signals.
- Invasive BCI targets mainly blind and paralyzed patients.

Disadvantages
- The main disadvantage is that invasive BCIs are prone to scar tissue build-up as the body reacts to a foreign object (electrodes) in the brain, causing the signal to become weaker.
- Surgery is risky and dangerous.
- It is not wireless.
- The process of conversation is slow.
- An invasive process is very expensive.

8.3.2 Partially Invasive BCI

Partially invasive BCI devices are implanted inside the skull, but rest outside the brain rather than within the gray matter. The system is illustrated in Fig. 8.4.

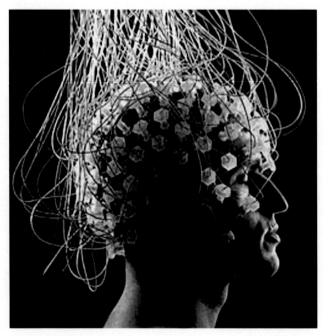

FIGURE 8.4   Example of partially invasive BCI.

Electrocorticography (ECoG) is an example of partially invasive BCI. ECoG provides brain signals that have an exceptionally high signal-to-noise ratio, less susceptibility to artifacts than noninvasive techniques, and high spatial and temporal resolution (<1 cm/<1 ms, respectively). ECoG involves measurement of electrical brain signals using electrodes that are implanted subdurally on the surface of the brain. Recent studies have shown that ECoG amplitudes in certain frequency bands carry substantial information about task-related activity, such as motor execution and planning, auditory processing, and visual-spatial attention. Most of this information is captured in the high gamma range (around 70–110 Hz). It has proven especially useful in advancing BCI technology for decoding a user's intentions to enhance and improve communication and control.[5]

Advantages
- Better quality of signal than noninvasive BCI.
- Partially invasive BCIs have less risk of scar tissue formation when compared to invasive BCI.

Disadvantages
- This approach typically results in a permanent hole in the skull.

8.3.3 Noninvasive BCI

Noninvasive BCIs rest outside the brain and try to capture brain signals (Fig. 8.5). Although the waves can still be detected, it is mote difficult to determine the area of the brain that created them and the actions of individual neurons. Noninvasive BCI produces poor signal resolution because the skull dampens signals, dispersing and blurring the electromagnetic waves created by the neurons. Signals recorded in this way have been used to power muscle implants and restore partial movement in an experimental volunteer.

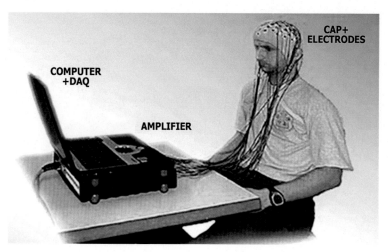

FIGURE 8.5   Example of noninvasive BCI.

Advantages

- It is applicable even in low quality signal.
- It is safest, as no surgery is required.
- Electroencephalography (EEG) is widely used for this technique.[6]

Disadvantages

- Muscle movement in noninvasive BCI can create artifacts.
- Noninvasive implants produce poor signal resolution.

8.4 BCI APPLICATIONS

8.4.1 Prosthetic Control

It is a well-known fact that the brain controls our actions and is the origin of all decisions, normally performed by modulating specific brain waves in the areas specialized for those tasks. In recent years BCI using EEG is emerging as a means to give communication and control.[7] EEG provides a medium for recording and accessing neural activity, thus facilitating computer retrieval and analysis of information from the brain signals produced by a thought. BCI research often focuses on finding a substitute for the broken mind–body chain that can help paralyzed patients move and communicate. The main purpose of BCI is converting a person's intent into action.[8,9] Thought-controlled arms, as shown in Fig. 8.6, are far from new, but an international team of researchers has apparently created an apparatus that aims to make the lives of paralyzed individuals easier. Though BCI application-oriented research has had beneficial results, including controlling wheelchairs, it uses expensive and bulky EEG equipment and highly skilled manpower. Technology is continuously getting smaller and cheaper, however, and recently several inexpensive consumer-grade devices have become available.

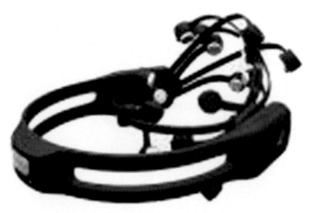

FIGURE 8.6   Emotive EPOC.

An example is the Emotiv EPOC,[10] a compact wireless headset that requires comparatively little effort to set up and allows much greater mobility than traditional EEG.

The EPOC was aimed at the gaming market, and is not classified as a medical device, though researchers have since adapted it for a variety of applications. The EPOC comes with processing tools that can detect facial movements, emotional states, and imagined motor movement. The last of these requires training for each individual to be able to control both the system and himself/herself. EPOC has 14 sensors arranged according to the international 10/20 system. The device has an internal sampling rate of 2048 Hz and, after filtering out artifacts, sends the data to the computer at approximately 128 Hz. These signals are transferred from the headset to the computer through wireless technology. This offers much greater mobility, and it is relatively simple to slip the headset on to the head. Instead of requiring a special gel, the electrodes of the EPOC simply need to be dampened using a saline solution, which is both disinfectant and common. There have been some applications that successfully utilize this technology, such as for identifying emotions and robot control.[11–13] An example is shown in Fig. 8.7.

The data collected by the headset is sent to the computer through an encrypted channel, and Emotiv supplies an application called EmoEngine to decode and process the data. This provides built-in brain-wave processing suites: Expressiv, which detects movement of facial features; Affective, giving a measure of five subjective emotions; and Cognitive, where users can train the system to detect specific thoughts. EmoEngine provides headset battery level, gyro readings, contact quality information, and researcher versions giving access to the raw EEG data. There is a C++ application program interface to allow custom applications using the supplied engine, and Emotiv gives examples of interfacing the engine using Java, .NET, and MatLab.

All of this functionality can be used without a custom application through the supplied control panel. The panel has a tab for each suite with a simple interface for visualizing and controlling it, along with a display of the contact quality of each sensor. Along with these

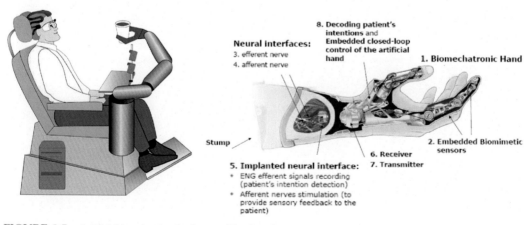

FIGURE 8.7 Artificial hand using brain–machine interface.

tools comes EmoKey, for mapping thoughts and expressions to keyboard input; EmoCube, a standalone version of the demonstration virtual cube seen in the control panel, which allows custom applications to utilize the moving cube visualization; and Testbench for researcher versions, which displays the electrode measurements and their Fast Fourier Transform, and allows recording of the data to disk.

8.4.2 BCI in Fatigue and Driver Alertness

Driver drowsiness is one of the major causes of serious traffic accidents. According to the National Highway Traffic Safety Administration (NHTSA),[14] there are about 56,000 crashes caused by drowsy drivers every year in India, which results in about 1550 fatalities and 40,000 nonfatal injuries annually. The actual tolls may be considerably higher than these statistics, since large numbers of driver-inattention accidents caused by drowsiness are not included in these numbers. The National Sleep Foundation also reported that 60% of adult drivers have driven while feeling drowsy in the past year, and 37% have actually fallen asleep at the wheel.[15] For this reason, a technique that can detect real-time driver drowsiness is of utmost importance to prevent drowsiness-caused accidents. If drowsiness status can be accurately detected, incidents can be prevented by countermeasures, such as arousing of the driver and deactivation of cruise control.

The sleep cycle is divided into no-rapid-eye-movement (NREM) sleep and rapid-eye-movement sleep, and NREM sleep is further divided into stages 1–4. Drowsiness is stage 1 of NREM sleep—the first stage of sleep.[16] A number of efforts have been reported in the literature on developing drowsiness detection systems for drivers. The NHTSA has also supported several research projects on driver drowsiness detection (Fig. 8.8).

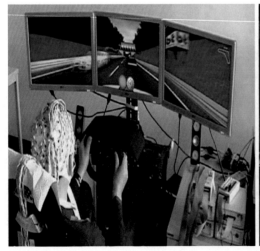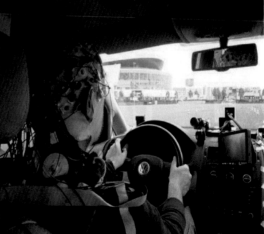

FIGURE 8.8   Examples of systems to recognize driver drowsiness.

Sleepiness in drivers has been identified as a causal component in numerous accidents, because of the marked decrease in drivers' view of danger and acknowledgment of threat, and their lessened capacities to take care of their vehicles. The National Sleep Foundation reported that 51% of adult drivers had driven a vehicle while feeling sleepy and 17% had really nodded off. Thus constant observation of sleepiness is critical to prevent car crashes. Past studies have proposed various techniques to recognize tiredness, which can be sorted into two fundamental methodologies. The main methodology concentrates on physical changes caused by exhaustion, such as the driver's slanted head, slumped body stance, and decreased holding power on the steering wheel. The driver's body changes are identified by direct sensor contacts or camcorders. Since these strategies permit noncontact discovery of sleepiness, they do not give the driver any distress. This increases the drivers alertness in utilizing the system. However, these parameters shift in diverse vehicle types and driving conditions. The second approach concentrates on measuring physiological changes of drivers, for example eye-action measures, pulse rate, skin electric potential, and EEG activity. A constant remote EEG-based BCI framework for fatigue identification is presented in Fig. 8.9.[17]

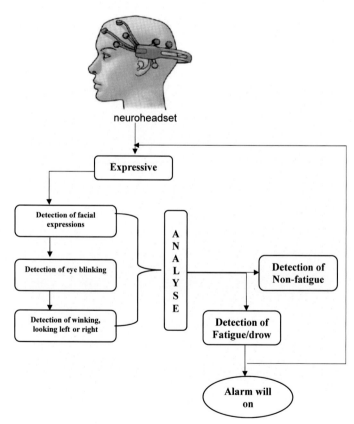

FIGURE 8.9   Outline of a real-time intelligent alarm system for driver fatigue based on the Emotive EPOC analysis system.

8.4.3 The P300 Speller[18]

A positive deflection in an EEG over the parietal cortex of about 300 ms is generated after infrequent stimuli. This response is termed the "P300" or "oddball" potential. Cz is the electrode around which the spatial amplitude distribution of P300 is centered. It is largest as the parietal electrode gets attenuated as the recording sites move to central and frontal locations.

Temporally, a typical P300 response has a width of 150–200 ms and a triangular shape. The peak potential of a P300 is typically 2–5 μV. Thus a single P300's signal-to-noise ratio is low, and is typically enhanced by averaging over multiple responses.

The P300 potential has been used as the basis for a BCI system in many studies. The classic format developed by Donchin and colleagues presents the user with a matrix of characters, as shown in Fig. 8.10.

The rows and columns in this matrix flash successively and randomly at a rapid rate (eg, eight flashes per second). The user selects a character by focusing attention on it and counting how many times it flashes. The row or column that contains this character evokes a P300 response (Fig. 8.11), whereas all others do not. After averaging several responses, the computer can determine the desired row and column (ie, the row/column with the highest P300 amplitude), and thus the desired character.

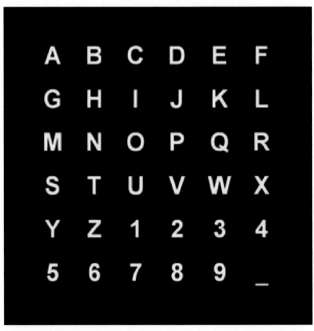

FIGURE 8.10   Character matrix of P300.

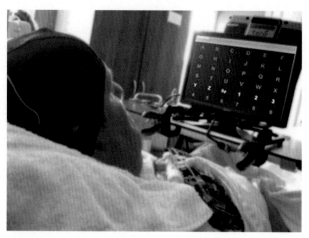

FIGURE 8.11   Example of subject with P300 speller.

8.4.3.1 *Characteristics of P300*
- The waveform is consistently detectable and elicited in response to precise stimuli.
- The P300 waveform can also be evoked in nearly all subjects with little variation in measurement techniques, which may help simplify interface designs and permit greater usability.
- The speed at which an interface is able to operate depends on how detectable the signal is despite "noise."
- The amplitude of the waveform requires averaging of multiple recordings to isolate the signal. This and other postrecording processing steps determine the overall speed of an interface.

8.4.3.2 *Applications of P300*
- Reading P300 brain waves can reveal forensic information related to terrorist attacks.
- This technology is very useful to disabled people, as the patient can communicate through the P300 speller.
- Permits control of home appliances with thoughts.

8.4.4 Brain Fingerprinting

Brain fingerprinting can be viewed as a modern, and more accurate, lie detection test. It helps us to identify whether a person is guilty or innocent. When someone commits a crime, it is stored in his/her memory. If the person is innocent, no such traces are seen in the memory. Brain fingerprinting is a test to identify whether the details are present in the memory or not.

To get the details used in brain fingerprinting, certain images of incidents are shown along with other stimuli. EEG sensors are used to record the response of the person's brain on seeing these images. The P300 is used as a measurement of response.[19]

However, the human brain is capable of generating as well as modifying thoughts. The solution to this modification problem is to record the person's response to the stimulus within fractions of a second. The response is recorded before the person can modify it, or even be aware of his/her own thoughts.

8.4.4.1 Brain Fingerprinting Applications
1. Detecting the record of a specific crime, terrorist act, or incident stored in the brain.
2. Military and foreign intelligence screening.
3. Criminal cases.
4. To detect symptoms of Alzheimer's disease, depression, and other mental disorders.
5. To detect forms of dementia, including neurological disorders.[20]

8.5 CHALLENGES FOR BCI

There are many challenges that face BCI when used in real-world tasks.[1]

1. Low BCI signal strength. Extracting signals from the brain is not an easy task. The signal strength is low, and in most cases signal amplification is required.
2. Data transfer rate (bandwidth). The best data transfer rate from a subject was three characters. The very low data transfer rate makes BCI applications suffer from fast response.
3. High error rate. Due to the low data transfer rate and low signal strength, there is a high error percentage. In addition, brain signals have very high variability. Therefore, the expected error rate is high.
4. Inaccurate signal classification. The brain has centers from which signals can be captured using electrodes, but classifying the captured signals suffers from high interference and inaccuracy. Many signal classification techniques are utilized, including recently proposed computational intelligence techniques.

8.6 CONCLUSION

This chapter discusses the concept of brain–computer interfaces. The working of BCI is shown in simple steps, building on material covered in the earlier chapters. The types of BCI are explained, plus the merits and demerits of each type: users may choose the appropriate BCI according to the application intended. The chapter also presents some nonmedical applications of BCI, which show that although communicating with the brain externally is difficult, it is not impossible. The chapter concludes by outlining some challenges for BCI which can be tackled by upcoming researchers in this field.

References

1. Ramadan RA, Refat S, Elshahed MA, Ali RA. Chapter 2-basics of brain computer interface. In: Hassanien AE, Azar AT, eds. *Brain-Computer Interfaces, Intelligent Systems Reference Library*. 74. Switzerland: Springer International Publishing; 2015. http://dx.doi.org/10.1007/978-3-319-10978-7-2.

2. Freeman B, et al., eds. *Brain—Computer Interfaces, The Frontiers Collection*. Berlin, Heidelberg: Springer-Verlag; 2010. http://dx.doi.org/10.1007/978-3-642-02091-9.

3. Birbaumer N, Cohen LG. Brain—computer interfaces: communication and restoration of movement in paralysis. *J Physiol*. 2007;579(3):621—636.

4. Nijholt A, Bos DPO, Reuderink B. Turning shortcomings into challenges: brain—computer interfaces for games. *Entertain Comput*. 2009;1:85—94.

5. Hill NJ, Gupta D, Brunner P, et al. Recording human electrocorticographic (ECoG) signals for neuroscientific research and real-time functional cortical mapping. *J Vis Exp*. June 26, 2012;64. pii: 3993. http://dx.doi.org/10.3791/3993.

6. https://www.mepits.com/tutorial/173/Electronics-Devices/BCI---Brain-Computer-Interface. Accessed 11.08.14.

7. Wolpaw JR, Birbaumer N, McFarland DJ, Pfurtscheller G, Vaughan TM. Brain-computer interfaces for communication and control. *Clin Neurophysiol*. 2002;113(6):767—791.

8. Pfurtscheller G, Muller-Putz G, Scherer R, Neuper C. Rehabilitation with brain-computer interface systems. *Computer*. October 2008;41:58—65.

9. Birbaumer N. Breaking the silence: brain computer interfaces (BCI) for communication and motor control. *Psychophysiology*. 2006;43(6):517—532.

10. http://www.emotiv.com.

11. Szafir D, Signorile R. An exploration of the utilization of electroencephalography and neural nets to control robots. In: *Human-Computer Interaction — Interact 2011*. 2011:186—194.

12. Thobbi A, Kadam R, Sheng W. Achieving remote presence using a humanoid robot controlled by a non-invasive BCI device. *Int J Artif Intell Mach Learn*. 2010;10:41—45.

13. Jacques M. *Development of a Multimodal Human-Computer Interface for the Control of a Mobile Robot* [Masters thesis]. University of Ottawa; 2012.

14. DOT Report HS-808-707. *NCSDR/NHTSA Expert Panel on Driver Fatigue and Sleepiness, Drowsy Driving and Automobile Crashes*. Washington, DC: NHTSA; 1998.

15. Rosekind MR. Underestimating the societal costs of impaired alertness: safety, health and productivity risks. *Sleep Med*. 2005;6:S21—S25.

16. Gackenbach J. *Sleep and Dreams: A Sourcebook*. New York: Garland; 1986.

17. Fatima N, Mubeen MA. A real time drowsiness detection system for safe driving. *Int J Adv Technol Innovation Res*. October 2014;06(09):910—918. ISSN: 2348-2370.

18. Donchin E, Spencer KM, Wijesinghe R. The mental prosthesis: assessing the speed of a P300-based brain—computer interface. *IEEE Trans Rehabil Eng*. June 2000;8(2).

19. Farwell L. Brain fingerprinting: detection of concealed information. In: Jamieson A, Moenssens AA, eds. *Wiley Encyclopedia of Forensic Science*. Chichester: John Wiley; June 16, 2014. http://dx.doi.org/10.1002/9780470061589.fsa1013.

20. *Brain Fingerprinting*. https://en.wikipedia.org/wiki/Brain_fingerprinting.

Index

Printed in the United States
By Bookmasters